ATLAS OF
ISCHEMIC
CLINICAL AND PATHOLOGIC ASPECTS # HEART
DISEASE

ATLAS OF
ISCHEMIC
CLINICAL AND PATHOLOGIC ASPECTS
HEART
DISEASE

Guest Editors

JAMES T. WILLERSON, M.D.

Edward Randall III Professor and Chairman, Department of Internal Medicine,
University of Texas Medical School at Houston; Medical Director and Chief of
Cardiology, Texas Heart Institute, St. Luke's Episcopal Hospital, Houston, Texas

JAY N. COHN, M.D.

Professor and Head, Cardiovascular Division, Department of Medicine, University of
Minnesota Medical School, Minneapolis, Minnesota

Editors

HISAO MANABE, M.D., D.M.Sc.

President Emeritus, National Cardiovascular Center; Professor Emeritus,
Osaka University, Osaka, Japan

CHIKAO YUTANI, M.D., Ph.D.

Director, Department of Pathology, National Cardiovascular Center, Osaka, Japan

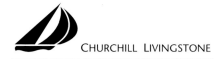
CHURCHILL LIVINGSTONE

New York, Edinburgh, London, Madrid, Melbourne, San Francisco, Tokyo

Library of Congress Cataloging-in-Publication Data

Kyoketsusei shin shikkan. English.
    Atlas of ischemic heart disease : clinical and pathologic aspects
/ guest editors, James T. Willerson, Jay N. Cohn ; editors, Hisao
Manabe, Chikao Yutani : with contributions by Chikao Yutani . . . [et
al.].
      p.   cm.
  Includes bibliographical references.
  ISBN 0-443-07924-2
  1. Coronary heart disease—Atlases.   I. Willerson, James T.,
Date.   II. Cohn, Jay N.   III. Title.
    [DNLM: 1. Myocardial Ischemia—atlases. WG 17k99a 1997a]
RC685.C6K96   1997
616.1′23—dc20
DNLM/DLC
for Library of Congress   96-29163
                                         CIP

Original Japanese edition published by Life Science Publishing Co., Ltd., Tokyo. English translation rights arranged through Churchill Livingstone Japan, Tokyo.

Distributed in the United Kingdom by Churchill Livingstone, Robert Stevenson House, 1–3 Baxter's Place, Leith Walk, Edinburgh EH1 3AF, and by associated companies, branches, and representatives throughout the world.

Medical knowledge is constantly changing. As new information becomes available, changes in treatment, procedures, equipment and the use of drugs become necessary. The editors/authors/contributors and the publishers have, as far as it is possible, taken care to ensure that the information given in this text is accurate and up to date. However, readers are strongly advised to confirm that the information, especially with regard to drug usage, complies with the latest legislation and standards of practice.

The Publishers have made every effort to trace the copyright holders for borrowed material. If they have inadvertently overlooked any, they will be pleased to make the necessary arrangements at the first opportunity.

Acquisitions Editor: *Allan Ross*
Assistant Editor: *Jennifer Hardy*
Production Editor: *Bridgett L. Dickinson*
Production Supervisor: *Laura Mosberg Cohen*
Electronic Publishing Coordinator: *Robb Quattro*
Cover Design: *Jeannette Jacobs*

Printed in Singapore

First published in 1997   7 6 5 4 3 2 1

Contributors

Chikao Yutani, M.D., Ph.D.
Director, Department of Pathology, National Cardiovascular Center, Osaka, Japan

Kazuo Haze, M.D., Ph.D.
Director, Department of Cardiology, Osaka City General Hospital, Osaka, Japan

Seiki Nagata, M.D., Ph.D.
Director, Department of Internal Medicine, Kansai Rousai Hospital, Hyogo, Japan

Tsunehiko Nishimura, M.D., Ph.D.
Professor and Director, Tracer Kinetics and Nuclear Medicine, Osaka University Medical School, Osaka, Japan

Masami Imakita, M.D., Ph.D.
Department of Pathology, National Cardiovascular Center, Osaka, Japan

Yoshitsugu Kito, M.D., Ph.D.
Vice President, Kinan General Hospital, Wakayama, Japan

Preface for the English Edition

This *Atlas of Ischemic Heart Disease* provides a thorough pictorial representation of coronary heart disease and its complications. A description of the anatomy of coronary arteries and of the process of atherosclerosis with detailed pictures is provided. Complications of coronary heart disease, including myocardial infarction, ventricular septal defects, ventricular aneurysms, rupture of the heart, and mitral insufficiency, are described and shown. The pictures included in the Atlas demonstrate representative electrocardiograms, echocardiograms, infarct-avid images, myocardial perfusion scintigrams, and postmortem findings. Topics such as coronary artery embolism, aortic dissection, percutaneous transluminal coronary angioplasty, intracoronary thrombolysis, and coronary artery bypass grafting are also discussed and demonstrated in detail. In short, the *Atlas of Ischemic Heart Disease* provides a detailed review of the anatomic, clinical, diagnostic testing, and complications of coronary heart disease, and it should be valuable for all who care for patients with coronary heart disease.

James T. Willerson, M.D.
Jay N. Cohn, M.D.

Foreword for the Japanese Edition

The "Color Atlas of Ischemic Heart Disease" is the second volume in a series, following the "Color Atlas of Valvular Heart Disease." In planning this series it was considered mandatory to provide pathologic and morphologic documentation for information obtained by various diagnostic techniques to ensure correct understanding and conceptualization of the disease.

Fortunately, abundant data resources on a wealth of patients, including over 10,000 surgical cases and more than 1,700 autopsies, were available at the National Cardiovascular Center. Such data enabled the successful publication of the first volume, "The Color Atlas of Valvular Heart Disease." At that time, the present work, "The Color Atlas of Ischemic Heart Disease," was planned as the next volume in the series.

"Ischemic Heart Disease" rather than "Myocardial Infarction" was selected as the title of this book because this policy provided for the inclusion of allied conditions, such as coronary arteriosclerosis and angina pectoris, as well as corresponding examples of patients undergoing diverse forms of internal and surgical therapy. In line with this policy, this publication presents classic examples of various forms of ischemic heart disease together with a dynamic combination of clinical and pathologic data.

However, as stated by the authors, the selection of a relatively simple disease entity such as ischemic heart disease created difficulty in the compilation of suitable clinical materials, owing to rather monotonous pictorial characteristics compared with valvular heart disease. Therefore, various forms of visual media were devised for this atlas, resulting in delicately detailed photographic plates, which may be described as being artistic, similar to the previous volume.

Ischemic heart disease, of course, accounts for a very high proportion of all cardiovascular disease. Moreover, the scope of cardiovascular disease is expanding, as exemplified by the recent inclusion of pediatric diseases such as Kawasaki disease. For physicians, internists, and surgeons alike, engaged in the diagnosis and treatment of cardiovascular disease, the 1980s witnessed major changes in both the pathology and therapy of ischemic heart disease. These changes are primarily attributed to successive advances made in defining the pathophysiology of ischemic heart disease, enabled through progress in basic research and diagnostic technology. Consequently, there has been a remarkable increase in the routine clinical use of techniques such as intracoronary thrombolysis (ICT) and percutaneous transluminal coronary angioplasty (PTCA) in internal medicine, and coronary artery bypass procedures in surgery. Recently, the use of left ventricular assist devices (LVAD) is also gradually increasing.

The present volume, dealing with the rapidly evolving pathology of ischemic heart disease, is thus unique in terms of its extremely novel, up-to-date content, providing the reader with a visual experience not possible through conventional textbooks and publications. I am therefore confident that this atlas will become a definitive text, unrivalled throughout the world, for the understanding of ischemic heart disease.

I sincerely hope that this book will be a valuable desk reference not only for specialists of cardiovascular disease, but also for physicians and researchers in all fields of medicine, as well as students aiming towards the future.

Finally, I would like to express my sincere gratitude to the effects of others who contributed to writing this book, especially Dr. Chikao Yutani, Director, Department of Pathology, National Cardiovascular Center who served as the senior editor. I also would like to thank Mr.Takaya of Life Science Publishing Co., Ltd., for his constant, deep understanding and cooperation in the publication of this book, and Mr. Takehara and Mr. Hatanaka of the editorial department of the company, as well as the photographer Mr. Kubo, for his continued effort in special photography.

Hisao Manabe, M.D., D.M.Sc.

Preface for the Japanese Edition

Over the past few years, numerous types of color atlases covering broad, diverse fields of medicine have been published in Europe and the United States. However, none of these publications have fully met the original aim of an atlas in providing "a faithful depiction of fact." For cardiovascular disease, the recent atlas by M. J. Davies and E. G. J. Olsen included rather small photographic plates, limiting the information that could be obtained from their perusal. The color atlas of A. E. Becker and R. H. Anderson is currently the best available, but there is still considerable room for improvement.

On being requested to serve as editor and author of a color atlas on cardiovascular diseases by Life Science Publishing Co., Ltd., our first thought was how to overcome the shortcomings of previous publications and produce the best color atlas yet.

The color atlas entitled "Valvular Heart Disease" was achieved through careful selection of appropriate cases from the wealth of patient documentation available, along with the concerted efforts of the editorial staff and photographers of Life Science Publishing Company. It is a remarkable atlas, the likeness of which had not been published previously. Our current work, "The Color Atlas of Ischemic Heart Disease," stems from our experience with that first atlas, and we are proud to state that it graphically depicts a brilliant world far beyond our expectations.

The clinical material for "Valvular Heart Disease" is intrinsically three-dimensional and shows marked visual diversity, whereas specimens for "Ischemic Heart Disease" are relatively one-dimensional and monotonous visually, making their compilation difficult. Therefore, considerable effort was required to present supporting material in the form of an atlas. For example, great care was exercised to reproduce the subtle color changes that reflect the time course of myocardial infarcts. Newly developed optical equipment was used to photograph sections of the entire myocardium allowing for the reproduction of delicate details. Sclerotic stenosis and thrombosis of the coronary arteries, which could formerly only be macroscopically visualized in transverse sections, were depicted longitudinally, whenever possible, to produce three-dimensional images.

Through these efforts, this atlas presents a more comprehensive review of the pathology of myocardial infarction than previous textbooks and atlases. It also includes the latest developments in the pathology and treatment of coronary arteriosclerosis and angina pectoris.

The rapid progress being made in the pathologic research, diagnosis, and treatment of ischemic heart disease may make this color atlas a 'classic' sooner or later. However, we edited this book fully aware that unforeseen obstacles may be encountered at any time when advancing into untrodden territory. There were instances where the authors could not reach agreement, even with regard to the most appropriate terminology. However, this was regarded as being currently unavoidable, but we must venture to say that inconsistencies may remain in the text, and welcome readers' criticism.

Finally, we would like to thank Dr. Kumiko Tanuma of the Department of Anatomy, Nippon Medical School, for kindly consenting to lend us the cast models of the coronary arteries.

Chikao Yutani
Kazuo Haze
Seiki Nagata
Tsunehiho Nishimura
Masami Imakita
Yoshitsugu Kito

Contents

I
General Aspects

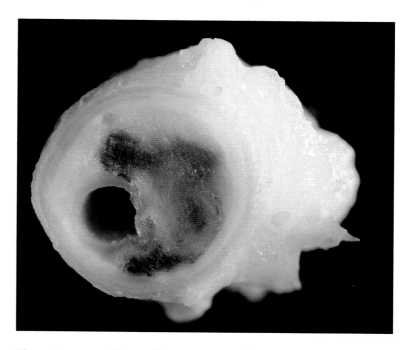

The patient was a 76-year-old woman. Seven days after an acute myocardial infarction, a ventricular septal rupture occurred, and the patient died about 1 month later. This photograph shows hemorrhage within an atheroma situated in the left anterior descending artery (segment 6). Thrombus formation was noted adjacently.

1. Coronary Arteries

Distribution of the Coronary Arteries

The ostia of the coronary arteries are situated in the left and right coronary artery sinuses (sinuses of Valsalva) lying adjacent to the aortic semilunar valve (Figs. 1, 2, and 3). The right conus artery is the first branch of the right coronary artery in about 50% of autopsies, but in the remaining 50%, it is an independent vessel referred to as the third coronary artery (Figs. 4 and 5). The ostium of this artery is typically adjacent to the right coronary artery orifices. Occasionally, the coronary artery ostia may extend beyond the border of the sinuses of Valsalva and the aortic wall (i.e., the sinotubular ridge) and thus exhibit "high takeoff" (Fig. 6).

RIGHT CORONARY ARTERY

The right coronary artery arises from the sinus of Valsalva and usually passes along the inferior surface of the right atrial appendage to the posterior or right atrioventricular groove toward the bundle branch (Fig. 7). The right coronary artery may bend transiently from the orifice or branch into the sinus node artery distal to the conus artery (Fig. 8). The conus artery is clinically significant because it arises directly from the aortic wall. Furthermore, in the event of proximal occlusion of the left anterior descending artery extending beyond the vessels supply-ing the conus, the anterior descending artery anastomoses with the conus artery, establishing a collateral circulation pathway (Vieussens' circle) to feed the region administered by the anterior descending artery.

The sinus node artery arises with a comparable frequency from the right coronary artery and the left circumflex artery. Clinically, this artery is important because it becomes the feeder vessel if the right coronary artery or the left circumflex artery is occluded proximally to the atrioventricular node artery. The sinus node artery runs posteriorly via the atrial septum to create an anastomosis between the atrioventricular node artery and the right coronary artery or the circumflex artery (Kugel's artery). Before arriving at the acute margin, the right coronary artery normally branches into two or three right ventricular arteries running perpendicularly. The branch that runs directly to the apex of the heart along the acute margin is known as the acute marginal artery. In the presence of severe stenosis of proximal portions of the posterior descending artery or anterior descending artery, the marginal branch anastomoses with the distal side of either of these arteries.

The classification of the American Heart Association (AHA) divides the right coronary artery into four segments: segment 1 refers to the proximal region up to the first right ventricular branch; segment 2 runs to the acute margin; segment 3 proceeds from the acute margin to the junction of the posterior descending artery and the posterolateral branch; and the remaining portion of the artery is segment 4 (Fig. 9).

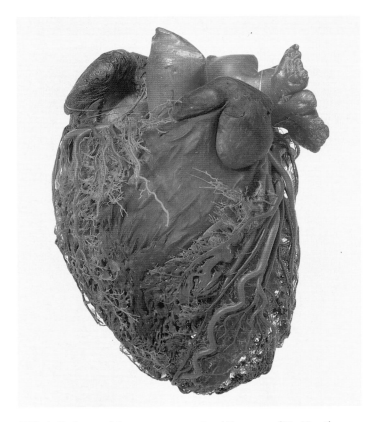
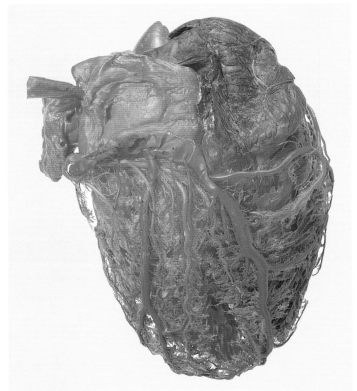

FIG. 1 Pathway of the coronary arteries. (Courtesy of Dr. Kumiko Tanuma, Department of Anatomy, Nippon Medical School.)

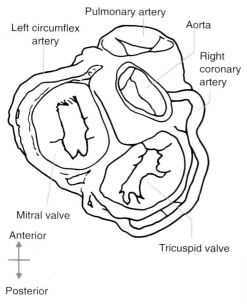

Pulmonary artery

Left circumflex artery

Aorta

Right coronary artery

Mitral valve

Anterior

Posterior

Tricuspid valve

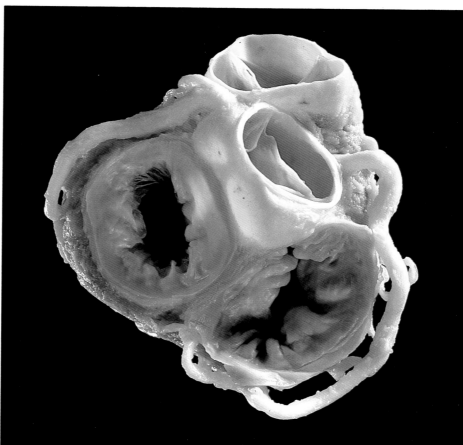

FIG. 2 Distribution of the coronary arteries. The distribution can be seen after the removal of the left and right atria.

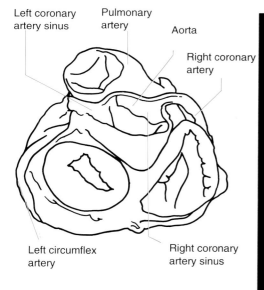

Left coronary artery sinus

Pulmonary artery

Aorta

Right coronary artery

Left circumflex artery

Right coronary artery sinus

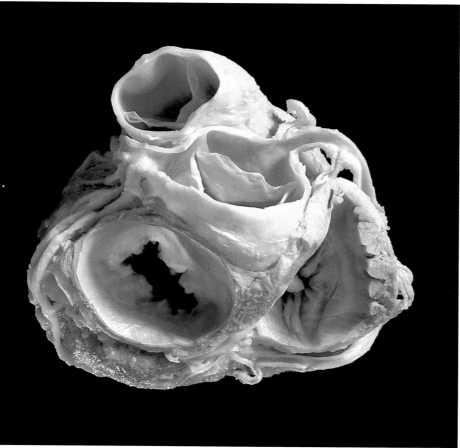

FIG. 3 Distribution of the coronary arteries. The arteries are seen arising from the sinuses of Valsalva.

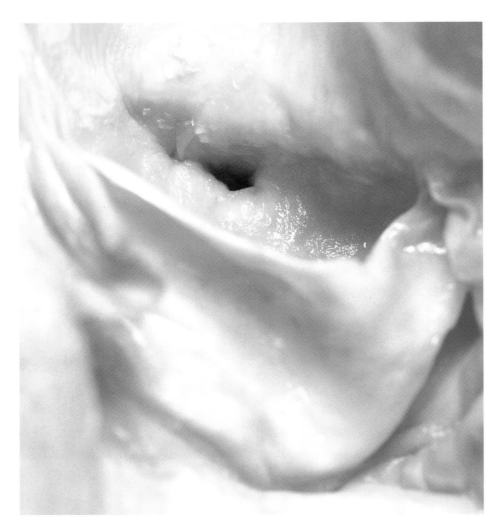

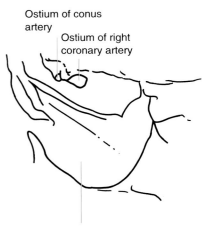

Ostium of conus artery

Ostium of right coronary artery

Right coronary cusp

FIG. 4 The conus artery arising separately from the right coronary artery.

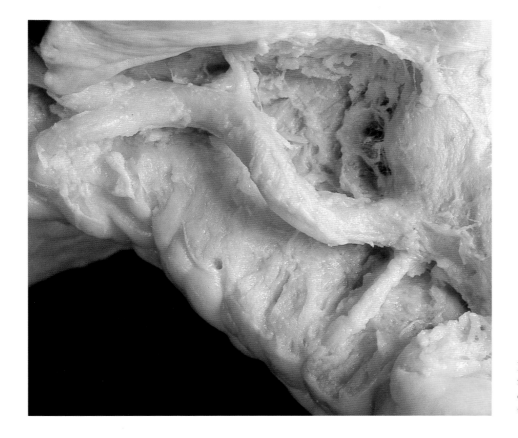

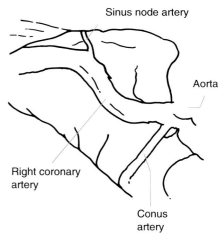

Sinus node artery

Aorta

Right coronary artery

Conus artery

FIG. 5 The conus artery arising separately from the right coronary artery. This is an epicardial view of the right coronary artery in the same patient as in Fig. 4.

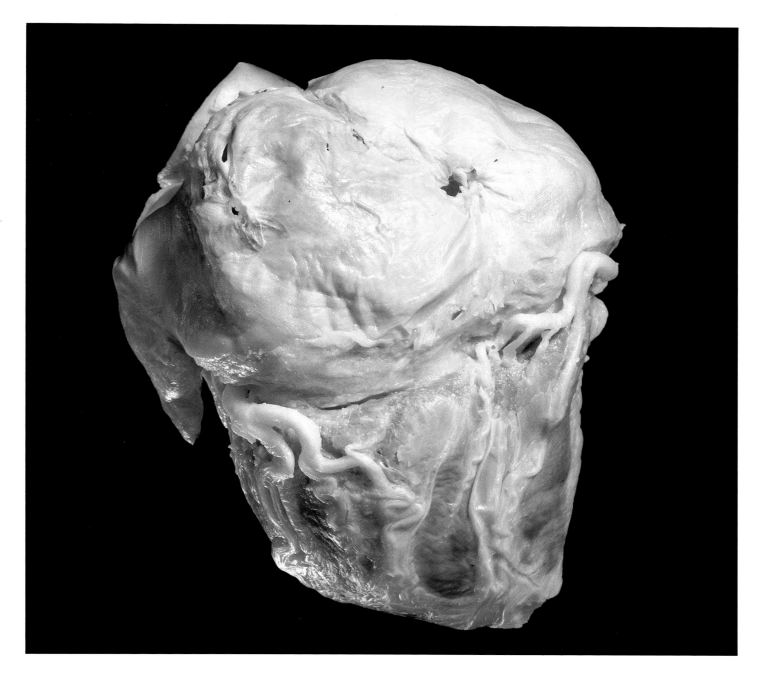

FIG. 11 Course of the left coronary artery (2). The anterior surface
(left page) and posterior surface (right page).

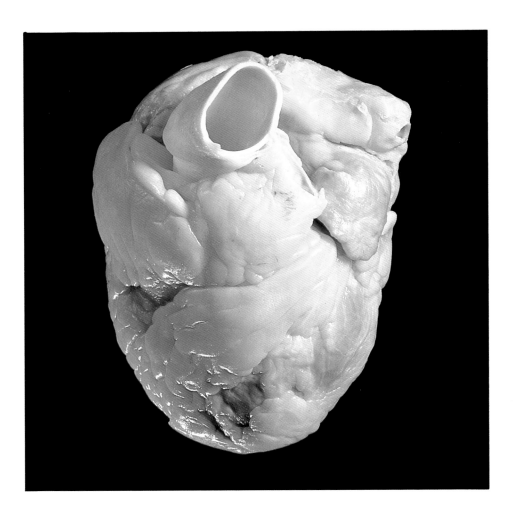

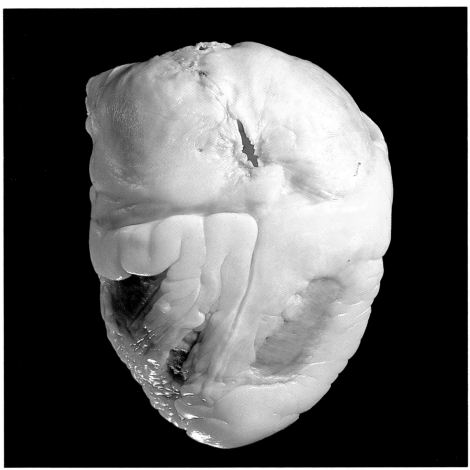

FIG. 12 Adipose tissue surrounding the coronary arteries, the anterior surface (top), and posterior surface (bottom) of the heart.

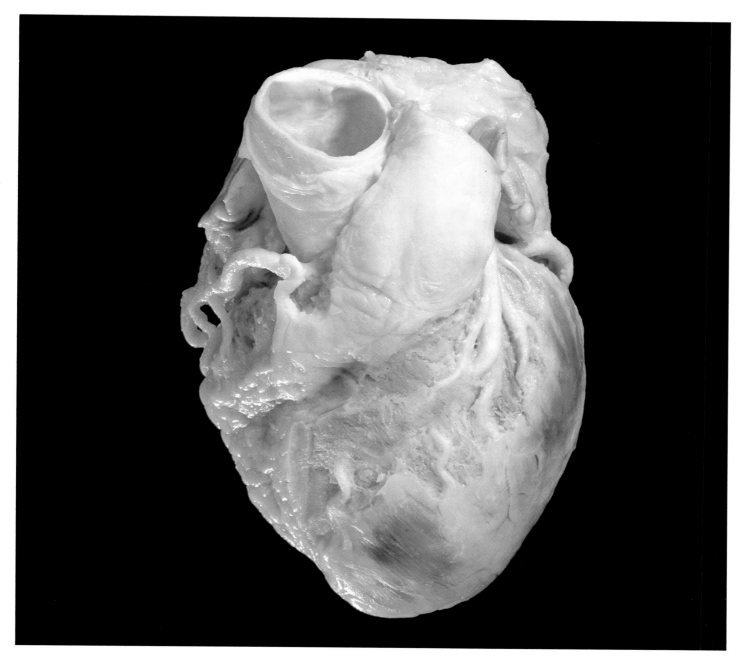

FIG. 13 A myocardial bridge. The left anterior descending artery runs intrapericardially after briefly running intramyocardially.

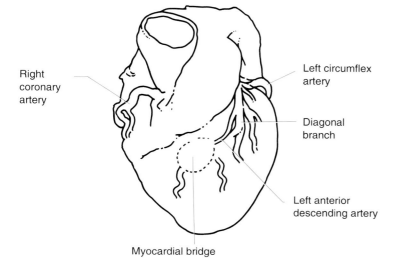

Right coronary artery

Left circumflex artery

Diagonal branch

Left anterior descending artery

Myocardial bridge

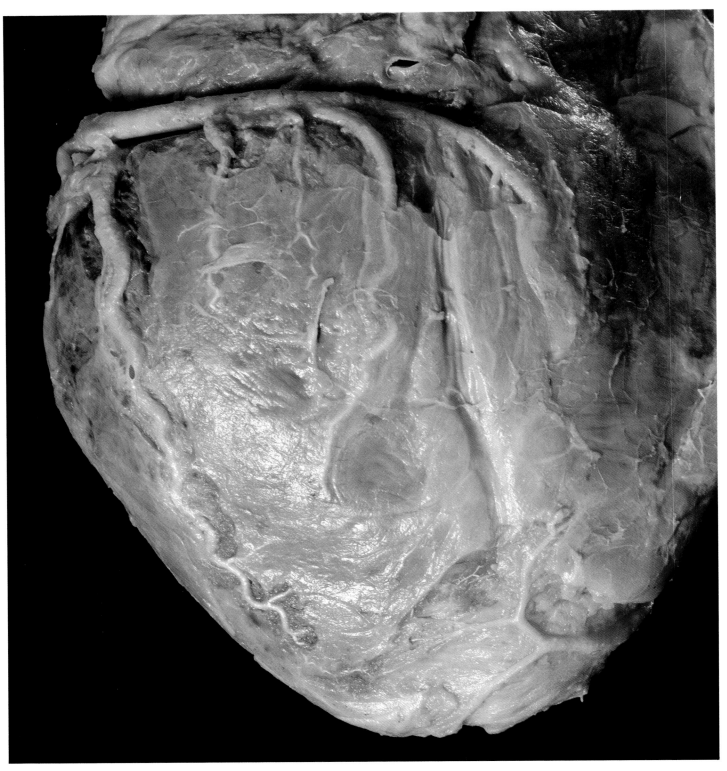

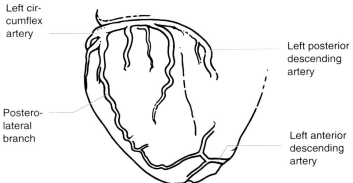

Left cir-
cumflex
artery

Left posterior
descending
artery

Postero-
lateral
branch

Left anterior
descending
artery

FIG. 14 Collateral circulation of the coronary arteries (1). An anastomosis between the posterolateral branch and the left anterior descending branch of the left circumflex artery can be noted. The right coronary artery is hypoplastic.

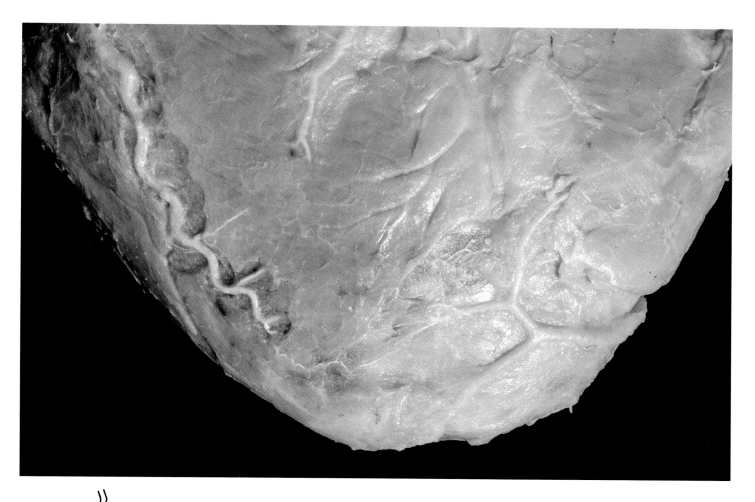

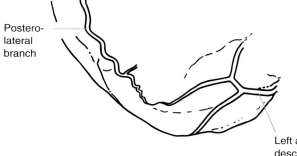

Postero-
lateral
branch

Left anterior
descending
artery

FIG. 15 Collateral circulation of the coronary arteries (2). An anastomosis between the left anterior descending artery and posterolateral
branch.

Coronary Artery Dominance

Appreciation of the region supplied by the coronary arteries is important to understanding the pathology of ischemic heart disease. This also applies when selecting the optimal therapeutic procedure, particularly in view of the recent increase in sophisticated techniques, such as intracoronary thrombolysis (ICT), percutaneous transluminal coronary angioplasty (PTCA), and coronary artery bypass grafting, as well as when assessing the patient's response to treatment and prognosis.

Schlesinger's rule, conventionally used to classify coronary artery dominance, assigns distribution patterns into three: right coronary artery dominance (type I), equal balance (type II), and left coronary artery dominance (type III). This system is both practical and easy to understand. Distribution patterns are classified into these types according to whether the right coronary artery or the left circumflex artery proceeds beyond the bundle branch (i.e., the intersection between the posterior atrioventricular sulcus and the posterior interventricular groove) and bifurcates into posterior descending branches.

Type I, in which the posterior (inferior) wall of the right ventricle, the posterior half of the ventricular septum, and the major portion of the inferior and posterior walls of the left ventricle are supplied by the right coronary artery, occurs in 48% of people (Fig. 16). Type II, in which the inferior wall (posterior wall) of the left ventricle is supplied by the left circumflex artery, is

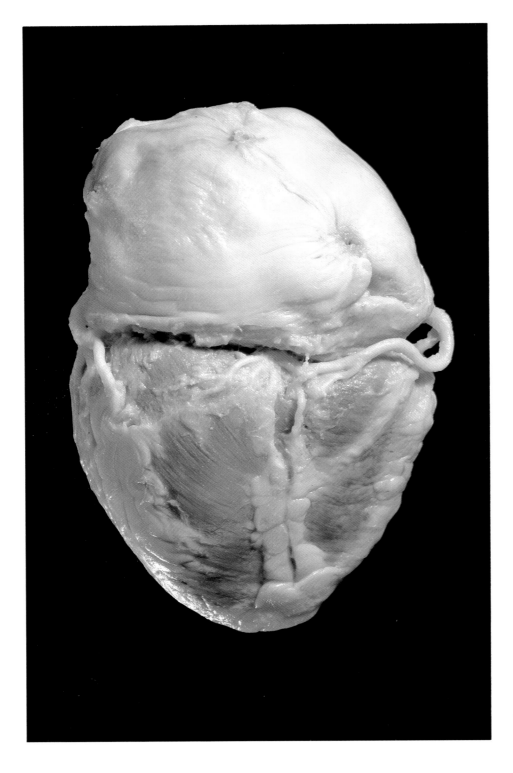

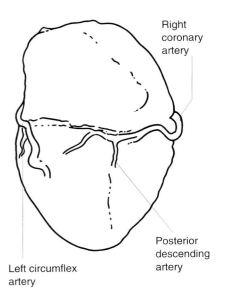

FIG. 16 Coronary artery distribution type (1). Right dominance.

noted in 34% of individuals (Fig. 17). Type III, in which the inferior (posterior) wall of the left ventricle, the ventricular septum, and the inferior (posterior) wall of the right ventricle are supplied by the left circumflex artery, and the posterior descending artery branches from the left circumflex artery, occurs in 18% of individuals (Fig. 18).

However, some investigators have proposed subtle differences in the criteria for defining coronary artery dominance. For example, some have recommended that dominance be defined on the basis of coronary angiographic findings indicating which regions are supplied by the left and right coronary arteries. In another classification system, proposed by Spalteholz, type II is defined by adjacency of the right coronary artery and left circumflex artery at the posterior wall of the left ventricle. Type I is characterized by the right coronary artery dominating the entire posterior wall of the left ventricle after bifurcating into posterior descending artery, with only a minor role played by the left coronary artery, and type III refers to the reverse situation.

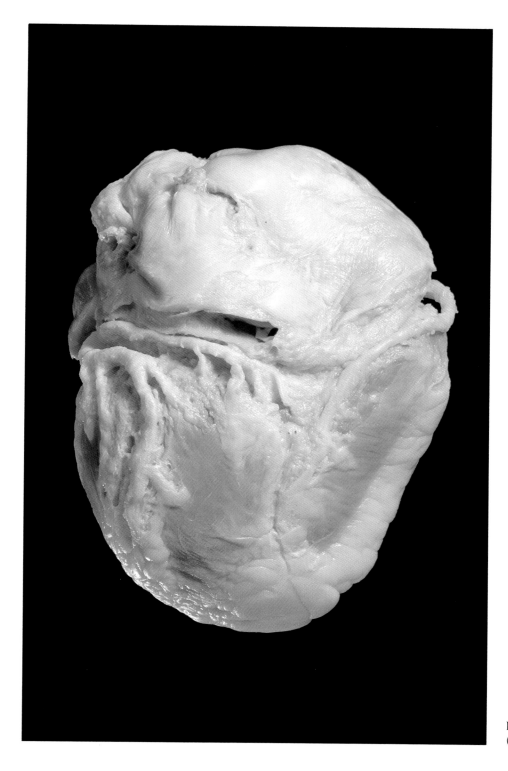

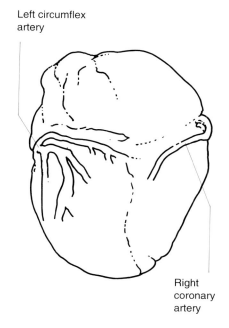

Left circumflex artery

Right coronary artery

FIG. 17 Coronary artery distribution type (2). Equally balanced.

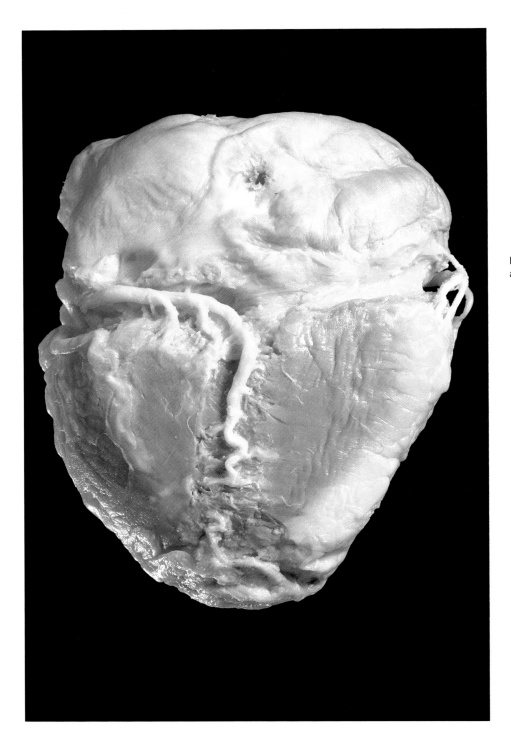

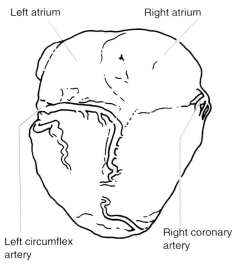

Left atrium

Right atrium

Left circumflex
artery

Right coronary
artery

FIG. 18 Coronary artery distribution type (3).
Left dominance.

2. Coronary Arteriosclerosis and Thrombosis

Coronary Arteriosclerosis and Thrombosis

Arteriosclerosis is a general term applied to localized arterial lesions producing thickening, hardening, and restructuring of the vascular wall. It can be broadly classified into atherosclerosis, occurring in large-size arteries (elastic arteries) and medium-size arteries (muscular arteries), and arteriolosclerosis, found in the arterioles. The term also includes mediosclerosis (Möncke-berg's sclerosis), principally associated with hyalinization, necrosis, and calcification of the media. Sclerosis of the arteries is essentially regarded as a physiologic aging phenomenon. However, a complex interplay of diverse factors is involved in the mechanism eliciting the onset and progression of arteriosclerosis. Historically, several theories have been proposed concerning the etiology of arteriosclerosis, including the thrombogenic theory of Von Rokitansky (1852) and Duguid et al. (1946), the plasma infiltration theory of Virchow (1862), the hyperlipidemia theory of Anitchkow (1913), and more recently, the monoclonal cell mutation theory of Benditt (1973) and the response to injury hypothesis of Ross et al. (1976). In addition to the vascular wall, arteriosclerosis can also affect the branching and course of blood vessels, as well as blood flow. Recently, regions of low shear stress have been reported to be particularly susceptible to atherosclerosis. Arteriosclerotic lesions also appear to be modified or accelerated by environmental, racial, genetic, and other factors, thus further complicating the onset and progression of arteriosclerosis.

INTIMAL THICKENING

The coronary arteries, which have a higher degree of diffuse intimal thickening than other arteries, are characterized by early signs of sclerosis, even in young subjects. Intimal thickening is generally caused by the proliferation of smooth muscle cells and an increase in extracellular matrices resulting from accumulation of mucopolysaccharides, connective tissue, and elastic fibers. The process of intimal thickening is associated with migration of smooth muscle cells from the media to the intima, as well as duplication and rupture of the internal elastic lamina.

Changes in the internal elastic lamina and intimal thickening start to appear in the coronary arteries soon after birth. Initial signs of intimal changes are already present at birth, and distinct thickening is noted in about 90% of infants from 1 month of age. Infants aged 3 to 4 months may have changes believed to be the initial lesions of arteriosclerosis, including degeneration and rupture of the internal elastic lamina, mucopolysaccharide deposition in the intima, and intimal cell proliferation.

This intimal thickening is regarded by some investigators to be a normal physiologic consequence of aging. Its high prevalence in arteries, in accordance with an increased likelihood of arteriosclerosis, suggests related involvement in the onset and development of this disease process.

ATHEROSCLEROSIS

Atherosclerosis of the coronary arteries is basically identical to atherosclerosis of other arteries. Focal sclerotic lesions are composed of cholesterol crystals, lipids, debris from cellular necrosis, connective tissue, mucopolysaccharides, lipophages, and smooth muscle cells. The atheroma surface is generally enclosed in an intimal connective tissue covering, referred to as the fibrous cap.

Two theories have been proposed to explain the origin of the foam cells, which characterize atherosclerosis. One suggests that they are medial smooth muscle cells that have migrated to the intima; the other suggests they are actually blood monocytes (macrophages) that have invaded under the endothelium.

Macrophages are mobilized initially for the dual purpose of phagocytizing and scavenging lipids deposited in the intima, but excessive phagocytosis occurs, leading to cell necrosis. Lysosomes are consequently released, initiating necrosis of the intimal connective tissue encapsulating the atheroma and promoting lysis of the atheroma itself. Further development of the atheroma is then accomplished through deposition of new thrombi and other substances. By contrast, extracellularly released lipids are phagocytized by smooth muscle cells, which promotes further atherogenesis.

Subsequent rupture of the atheroma and epithelial cell injury produced by hemodynamic and other factors result in thrombus formation, organization, and incorporation into the atheroma. During the process of thrombus organization, the coronary artery undergoes neovascularization, leading to edema and swelling of the atheroma associated with increased permeability. Perivascular inflammatory cell infiltration causes softening of the atheroma, and attendant factors such as lipid deposition and hemorrhage lead to either expansion or destruction of the atheroma. As a result of this vicious circle, stenosis of the coronary artery lumen progresses to occlusion.

The media at the site of arteriosclerotic lesions tend to be thin and fibrous. The adventitia likewise undergoes fibrosis and may display focal accumulations of chronic inflammatory cells, including lymphocytes and plasma cells.

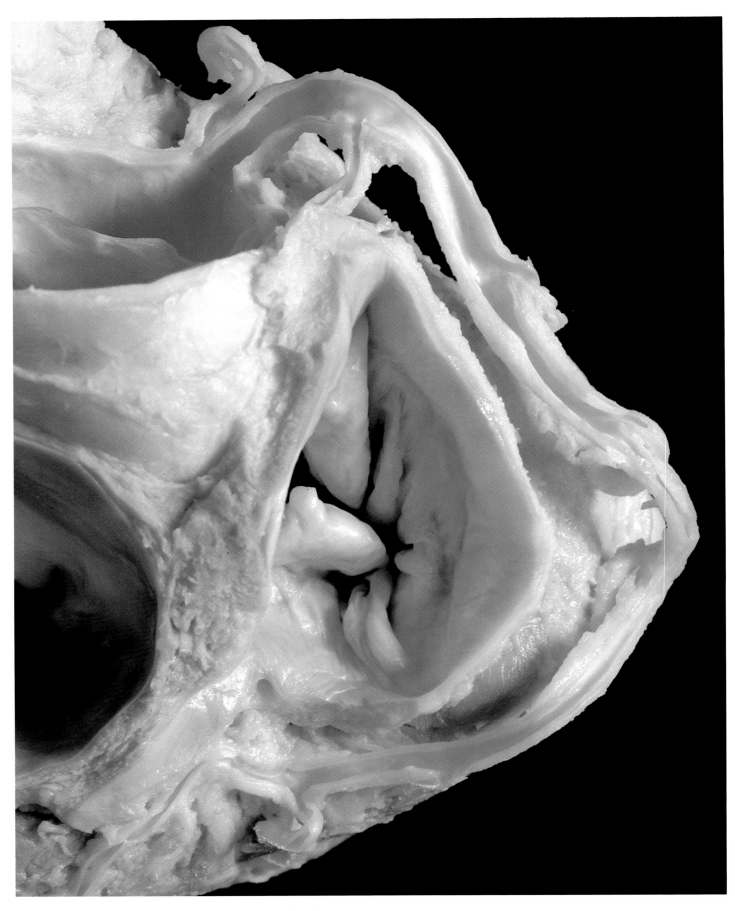

FIG. 19 Distribution of coronary arteriosclerosis (1) in the right coronary artery. Fibrous thickening and yellow plaques can be seen near the junction of the right ventricular artery and the branch leading to the sinus node.

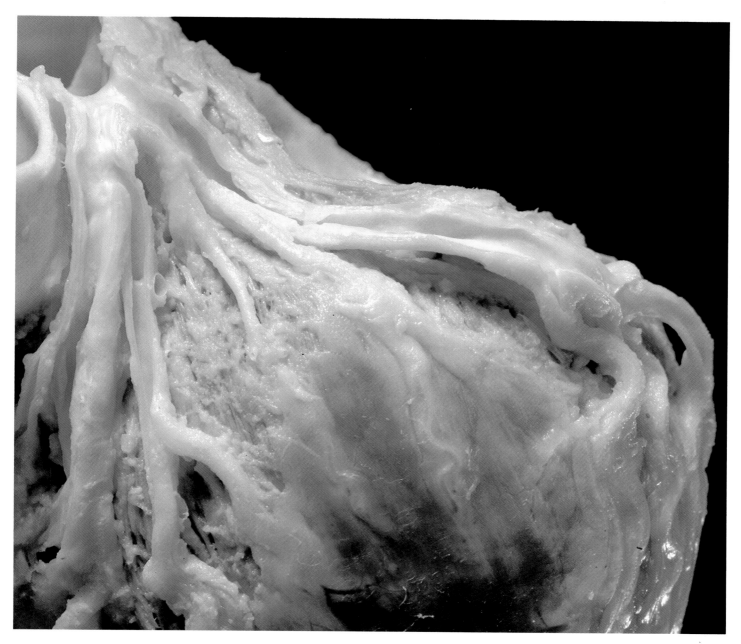

FIG. 20 Distribution of coronary arteriosclerosis (2) in the left coronary artery. Fibrous thickening and yellow plaques can be seen near
the junction of the left anterior descending artery and the left circumflex artery.

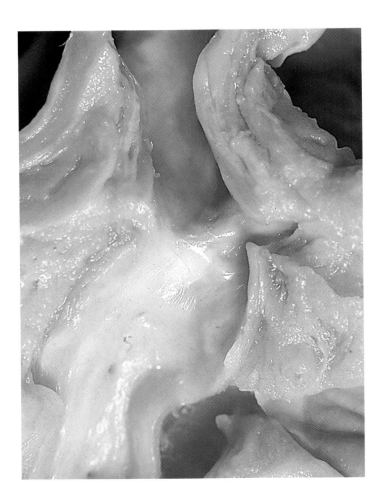

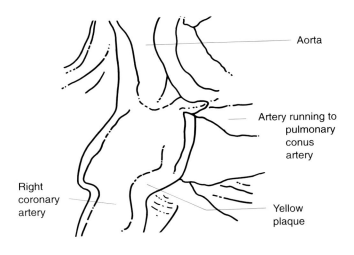

FIG. 21 Yellow plaques in the right coronary artery.

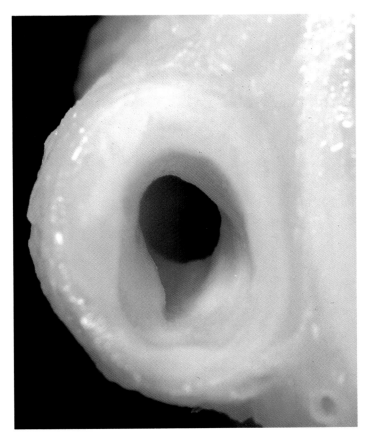

FIG. 22 Lumen of the right coronary artery. Unevenness resulting from fibrous thickening can be seen.

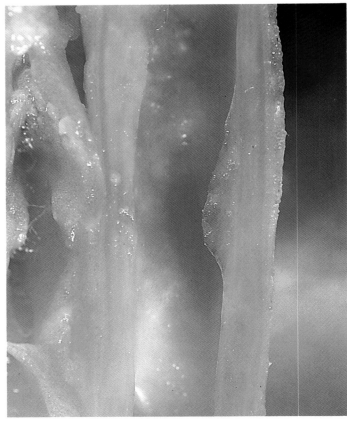

FIG. 23 Longitudinal section of the right coronary artery. Fibrous thickening associated with an atheroma can be seen in the intima.

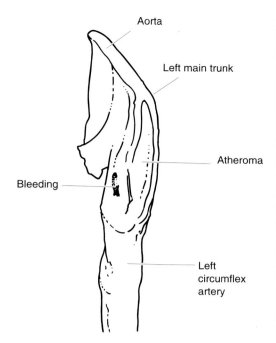

Aorta

Left main trunk

Atheroma

Bleeding

Left
circumflex
artery

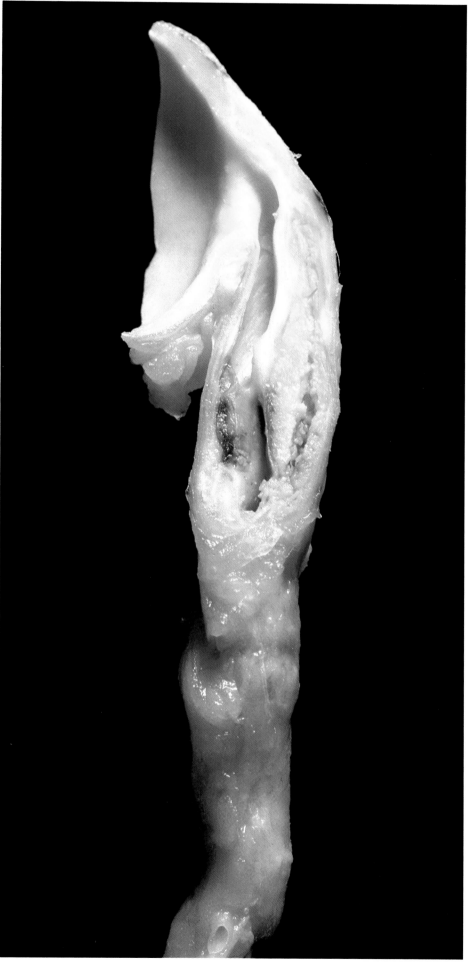

FIG. 24 Arteriosclerotic lesions of the
left main trunk.

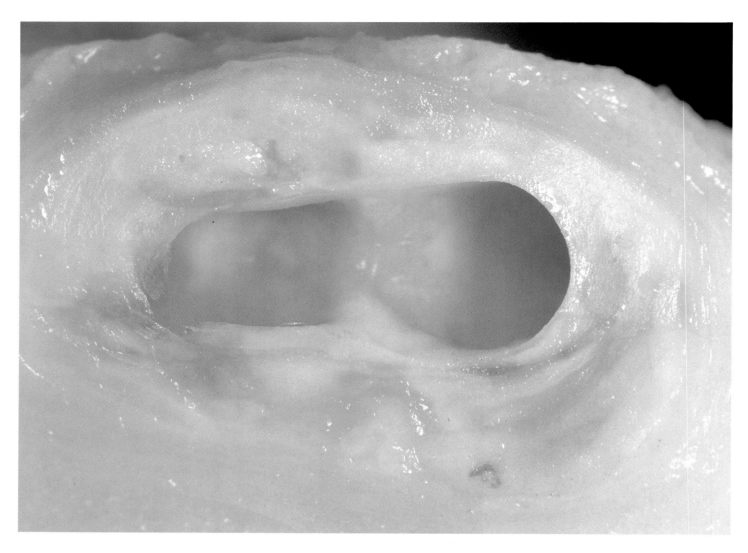

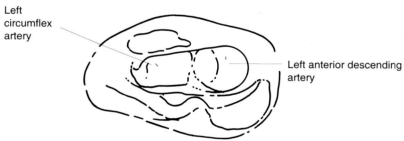

Left circumflex artery

Left anterior descending artery

FIG. 25 Junction of the left anterior descending artery and the left circumflex artery. Yellow plaques are evident on the intimal surface after bifurcation. An atheroma can even be seen in a section at the point of juncture.

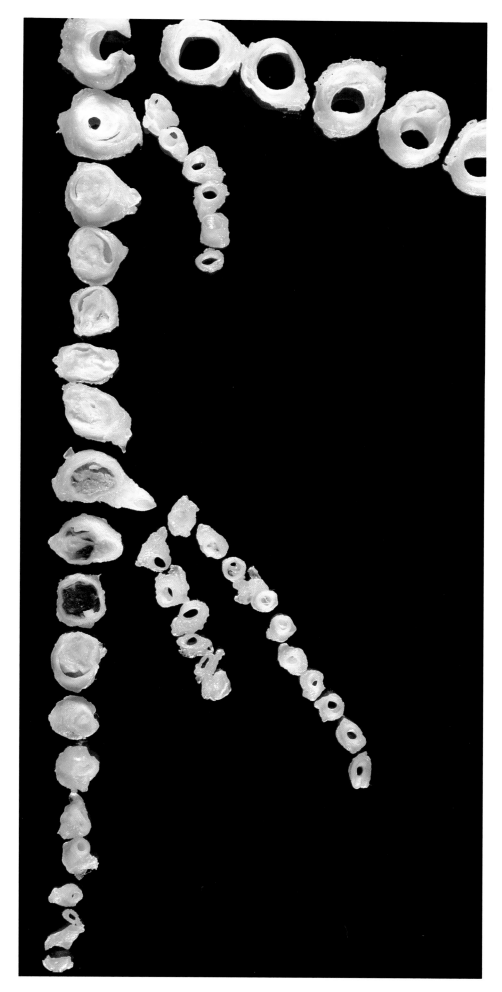

FIG. 26 Arteriosclerosis of the left anterior descending artery (1). Diverse lesions accompany complete occlusion of the left anterior descending artery.

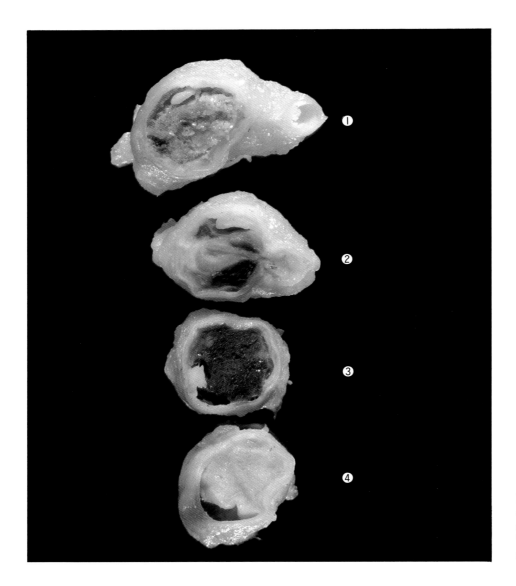

FIG. 27 Arteriosclerosis of the left anterior descending artery (2). From the top, a marked atheroma, occlusion by an organized thrombus, bleeding within the atheroma, and recanalization are presented.

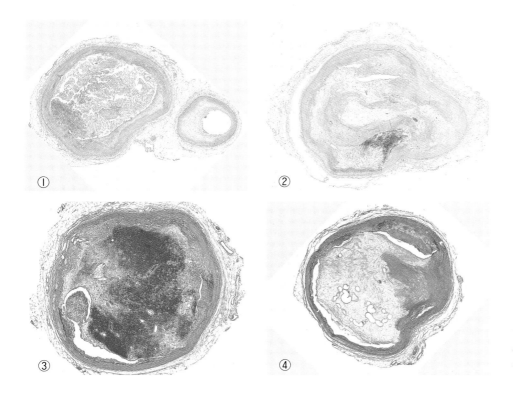

FIG. 28 Arteriosclerosis of the left anterior descending artery (3). Histologic findings associated with Fig. 27.

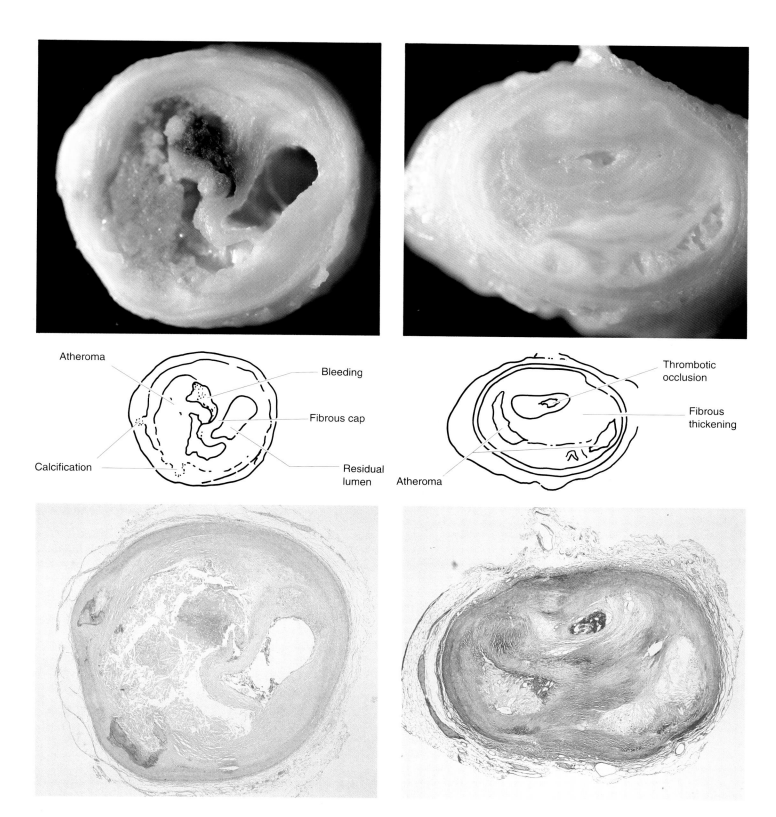

Atheroma

Bleeding

Fibrous cap

Calcification

Residual
lumen

Thrombotic
occlusion

Fibrous
thickening

Atheroma

FIG. 29 Coronary arteriosclerosis.

FIG. 30 Coronary arteriosclerosis.

CORONARY THROMBOSIS

Pathologic studies of myocardial infarction at autopsy and coronary arteriograms taken at the onset of infarction have frequently detected thrombi at sites of organized stenosis. Thrombosis thus appears to play a key role in the onset of myocardial infarction. By contrast, a clinical diagnosis of myocardial infarction is often unaccompanied by signs of thrombosis at autopsy or, conversely, insufficient clinical evidence to establish a definitive diagnosis of myocardial infarction may be associated with various signs of myocardial necrosis. Therefore, the opinion also exists that coronary thrombosis is secondary to myocardial infarction. In addition, coronary thrombosis has been confirmed in sudden death (myocardial infarction followed by death within 6 hours after onset) and in some patients with unstable angina pectoris. Thrombosis thus represents a major etiologic factor in ischemic heart disease.

Thrombi are classified as being either occlusive or mural, depending on whether the area occupied by the thrombus is equivalent to more or less than 50% of the residual lumen (Fig. 31).

The age of a thrombus may be estimated from the following morphologic characteristics to facilitate understanding the time course of thrombus formation (Figs. 32–41).

Fresh: Morphologically intact platelets, erythrocytes, and leukocytes entrapped in a fibrin network (within about 2 days).

Recent: The fibrin network becomes more densely stained than when in the fresh state; leukocytes and other cellular components undergo rupture and concentration, resulting in a uniform consistency (within about 6 to 7 days).

Organizing: Spindle-shaped cells appear in the thrombus and recanalization is evident (within 2 to 3 weeks).

Organized: An organized blood thrombus accompanied by recanalization (more than 3 weeks).

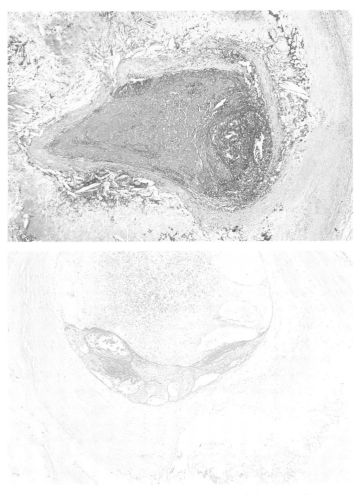

FIG. 31 An occlusive thrombus (top) and mural thrombus (bottom) of the coronary artery. (Top: Masson trichrome stain, × 25; bottom: HE stain, × 25.)

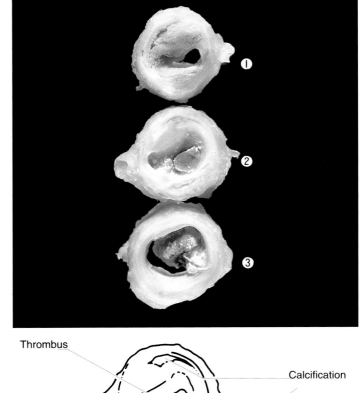

FIG. 32 Coronary thrombosis (fresh) (1). The lower part of the figure is a diagrammatic representation of photograph (2).

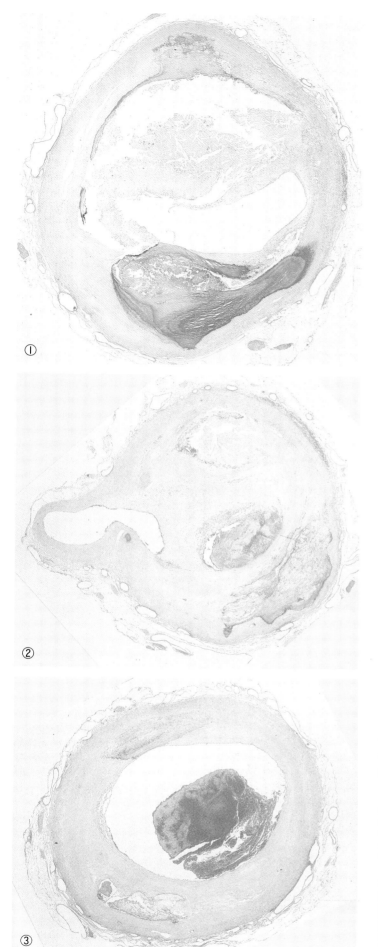

①

②

③

FIG. 33 Coronary thrombosis (fresh) (2). Histologic findings associated with Fig. 32. (HE stain.)

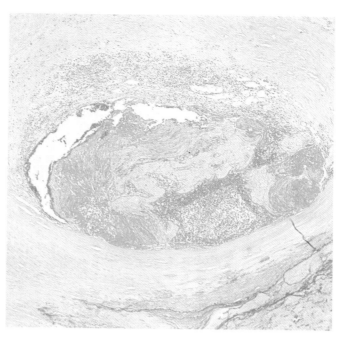

FIG. 34 Coronary thrombosis (fresh) (3). Close-up of the thrombus shown in Fig. 33 (2). (HE stain, × 30.)

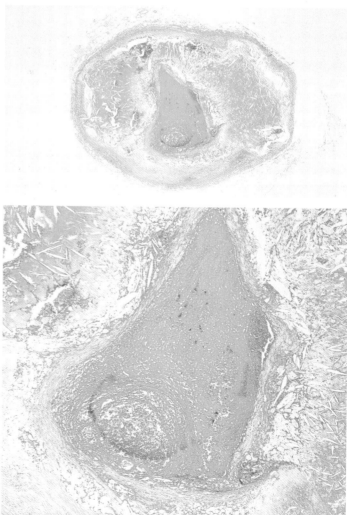

FIG. 35 Coronary thrombosis (recent). (HE stain, × 30.)

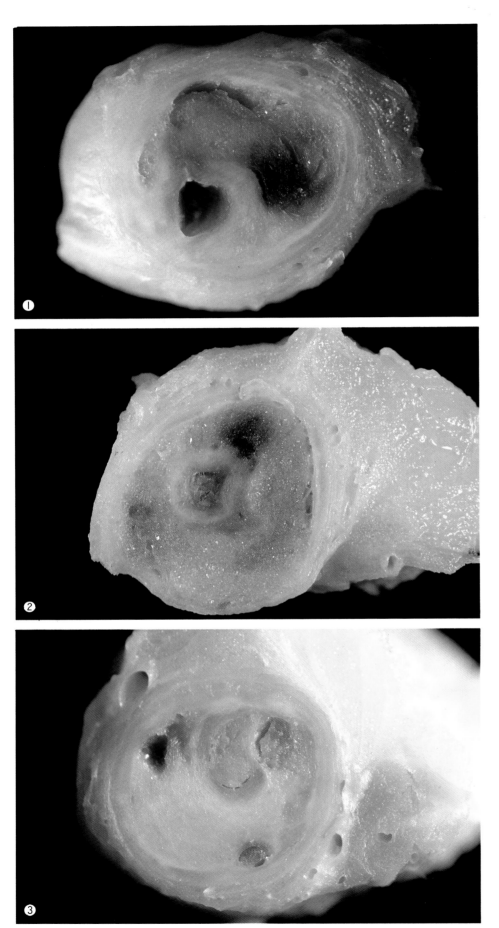

FIG. 36 Coronary thrombosis (organizing) (1). Serial sections.

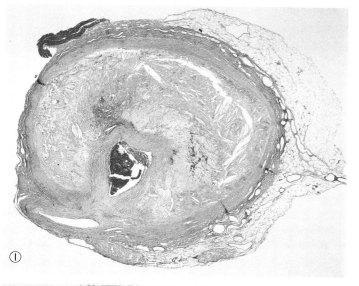

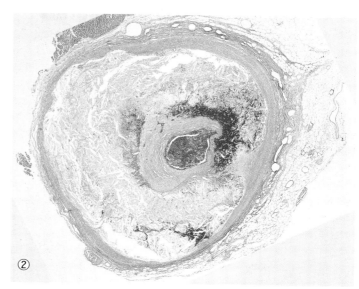

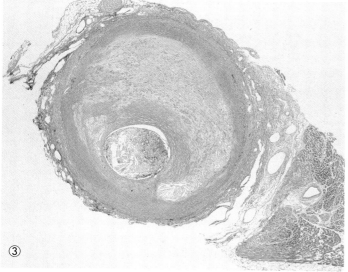

FIG. 37 Coronary thrombosis (organizing) (2). Histologic findings associated with the serial sections shown in Fig. 36. (Masson trichrome stain.)

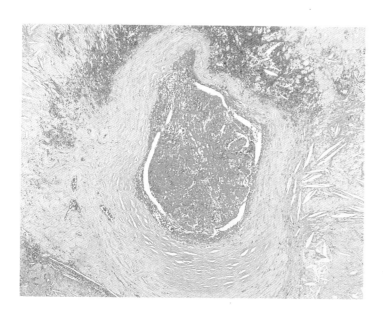

FIG. 38 Coronary thrombosis (organizing) (3). Close-up of the thrombus shown in Fig. 37. (HE stain, × 30.)

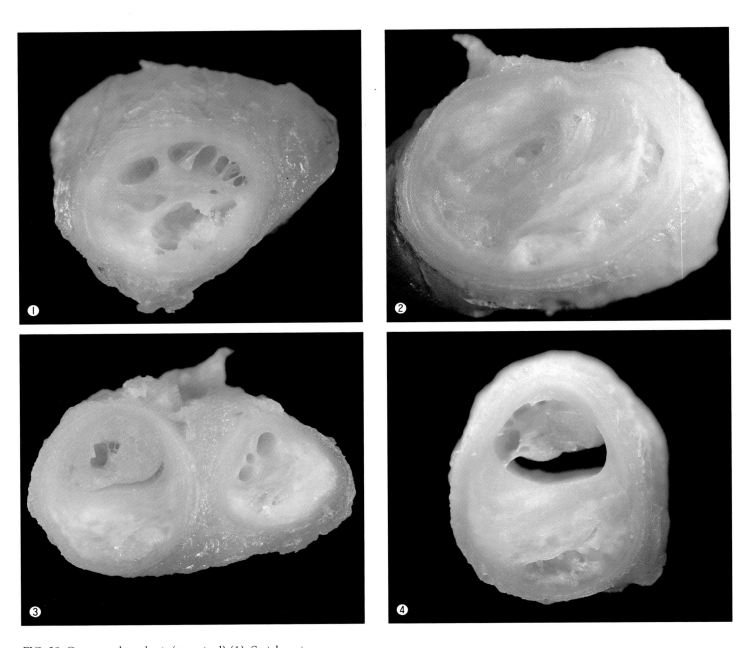

FIG. 39 Coronary thrombosis (organized) (1). Serial sections.

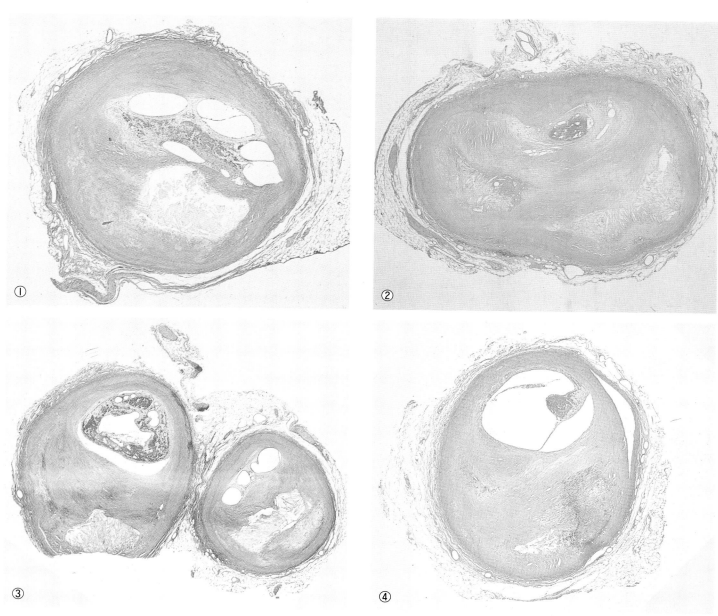

FIG. 40 Coronary thrombosis (organized) (2). Histologic findings associated with the serial sections shown in Fig. 39. [(1) and (3), Masson trichrome stain; (2) and (4), HE stain.]

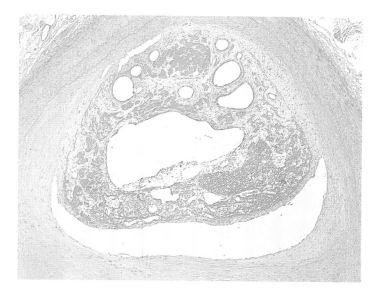

FIG. 41 Coronary thrombosis (organized) (3). Magnification of the thrombus shown in Fig. 40 (3). (HE stain, × 25.)

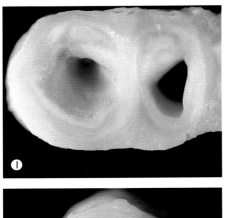

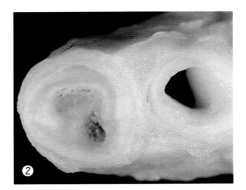

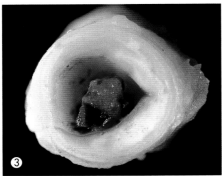

FIG. 42 Coronary thrombosis. Serial transverse sections taken at 3 mm intervals from just after the junction of the left anterior descending artery and the first diagonal branch. Formation of a thrombus, developing distally, is evident adjacent to the region of most marked stenosis caused by an atheroma.

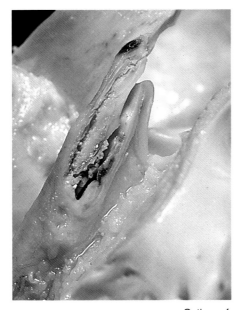

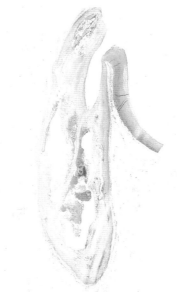

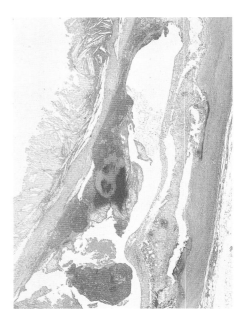

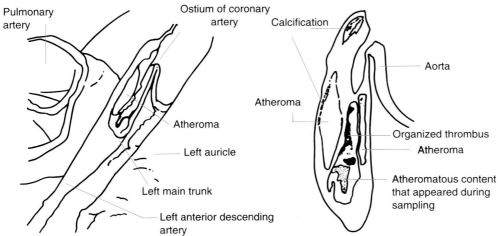

Pulmonary artery

Ostium of coronary artery

Atheroma

Left auricle

Left main trunk

Left anterior descending artery

Calcification

Aorta

Atheroma

Organized thrombus

Atheroma

Atheromatous content that appeared during sampling

FIG. 43 Coronary thrombosis.

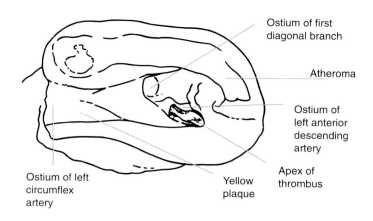

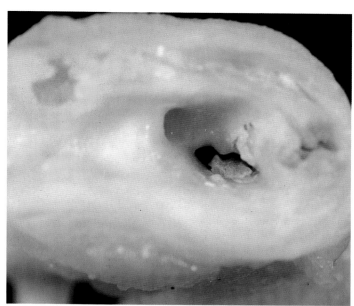

FIG. 44 Coronary thrombosis. Transverse section of the bifurcation of the left anterior descending artery and the left circumflex artery. The apex of a thrombus formed in the left anterior descending artery can be seen.

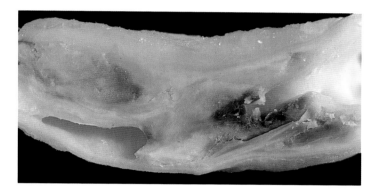

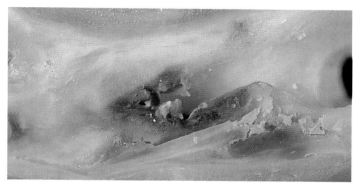

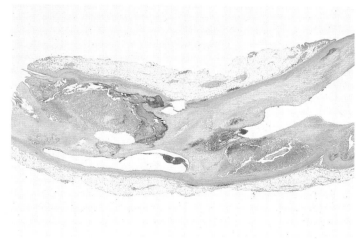

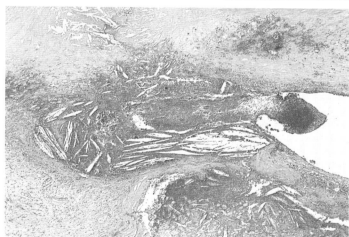

FIG. 45 Coronary thrombosis. Longitudinal section of the left anterior descending artery of the same patient as in Fig. 44. Rupture of the atheroma and thrombi is evident. The right side is proximal. (HE stain, × 25.)

Coronary Angiography

Coronary angiography, together with noninvasive methods such as the case history, clinical signs and symptoms, blood chemistry, electrocardiography (ECG), echocardiography, the Doppler method, and nuclear medicine examinations, is essential for the diagnosis, evaluation of severity, selection of treatment, evaluation of therapeutic efficacy, and estimation of the prognosis of ischemic heart disease. A detailed understanding of the presence, site, severity, and morphology of any coronary artery lesion can be obtained from coronary angiography. A dramatic improvement in safety, coupled with the increasing use of intracoronary thrombolysis (ICT) and percutaneous transluminal coronary angioplasty (PTCA), have made coronary angiography an important tool in both the diagnosis and treatment of ischemic heart disease.

INDICATIONS

Generally, the indications for invasive examination procedures depend on their necessity and safety. The indications for coronary angiography have been broadened significantly because of the increasing incidence of ischemic heart disease, improved safety of the procedure itself, and the increased use of therapies such as ICT and PTCA. The following patients are candidates for coronary angiography:

1. Patients with definite or probable ischemic heart disease: coronary angiography was initially contraindicated in acute myocardial infarction, but it is now actively used to assist ICT.
2. Patients over 50 years of age with valvular heart disease and patients with congenital heart defects indicated for surgery: coronary angiography is performed as a screening examination for coronary artery disease in the assessment of the underlying disease.
3. Patients with ECG abnormalities of unknown origin or heart failure.
4. Patients after coronary bypass surgery: confirmation of bypass patency.
5. Patients with Kawasaki disease: regardless of whether symptoms are present, because of the high concurrent incidence of coronary artery disease.

CONTRAINDICATIONS

1. Facility contraindications: facilities with a high incidence of complications and facilities that cannot obtain images that permit accurate evaluation of lesions for diagnosis.
2. Patient contraindications: patients with severe hypersensitivity to iodine. In the presence of ischemic attacks resistant to drug therapy, coronary angiography is now indicated even for elderly patients, patients with marked motor function disturbances resulting from cerebrovascular disease, and patients with advanced cancer, because of the availability of PTCA as a therapeutic procedure.
3. Temporal contraindications: the active phase of infections, including myocarditis and 2 to 3 hours after meals. In infections, the patient's condition may be aggravated, hampering the treatment of any complications, and emergency surgery cannot be performed even when required on the basis of the results of examinations. Coronary angiography after meals is dangerous because of the risk of vomiting during the procedure.

METHODS

1. Percutaneous femoral artery puncture: this method uses two catheters, designed to facilitate insertion into the orifices of the left and right coronary arteries. Judkins, Amplatz, and Bourassa catheters are used. A different catheter type is required for left ventriculography.
2. Brachiocephalic artery incision: bilateral coronary angiography and left ventriculography are performed using a single catheter. Although this can also be accomplished by femoral artery puncture using a single multipurpose catheter, catheter maneuverability is often hampered by tissue resistance at the puncture site or sheath valve resistance.

The technique of brachiocephalic artery incision has not undergone any major revisions over the last 30 years. The development of thin flexible catheters (5 F) for femoral artery puncture has enhanced safety and shortened the subsequent period of bed rest. However, a certain degree of technical competence in the brachiocephalic artery incision technique is necessary to cope with situations that preclude execution of femoral artery puncture.

COMPLICATIONS

Etiology: various complications may be caused by arteriotomy, puncture, catheter manipulation, and other procedural techniques, as well as by the contrast media. The incidence of complications is relatively high in more serious cases, such as those involving left main trunk lesions and marked left ventricular dysfunction.

NORMAL CORONARY ANGIOGRAMS

Figures 46 to 48 show the names of the normal coronary arteries, arteriograms, and resin specimens positioned isotopically to the angiograms.

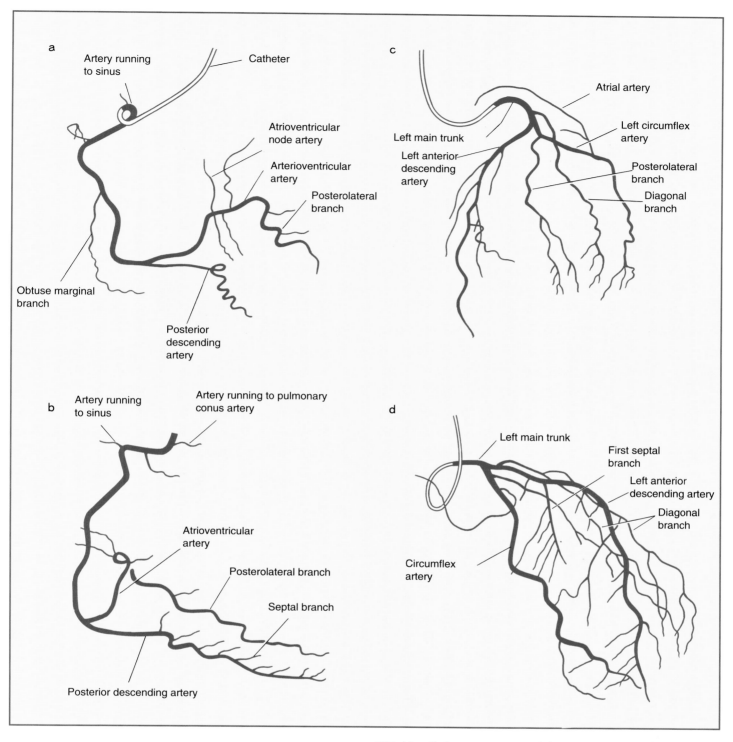

a

Artery running
to sinus

Catheter

Atrioventricular
node artery

Arterioventricular
artery

Posterolateral
branch

Obtuse marginal
branch

Posterior
descending
artery

c

Atrial artery

Left main trunk

Left circumflex
artery

Left anterior
descending
artery

Posterolateral
branch

Diagonal
branch

b

Artery running
to sinus

Artery running to pulmonary
conus artery

Atrioventricular
artery

Posterolateral branch

Septal branch

Posterior descending artery

d

Left main trunk

First septal
branch

Left anterior
descending artery

Diagonal
branch

Circumflex
artery

FIG. 46 a: Right coronary artery, left anterior oblique view; b: right coronary artery, right anterior oblique aspect; c: left coronary artery, left anterior oblique aspect; d: left coronary artery, right anterior oblique view.

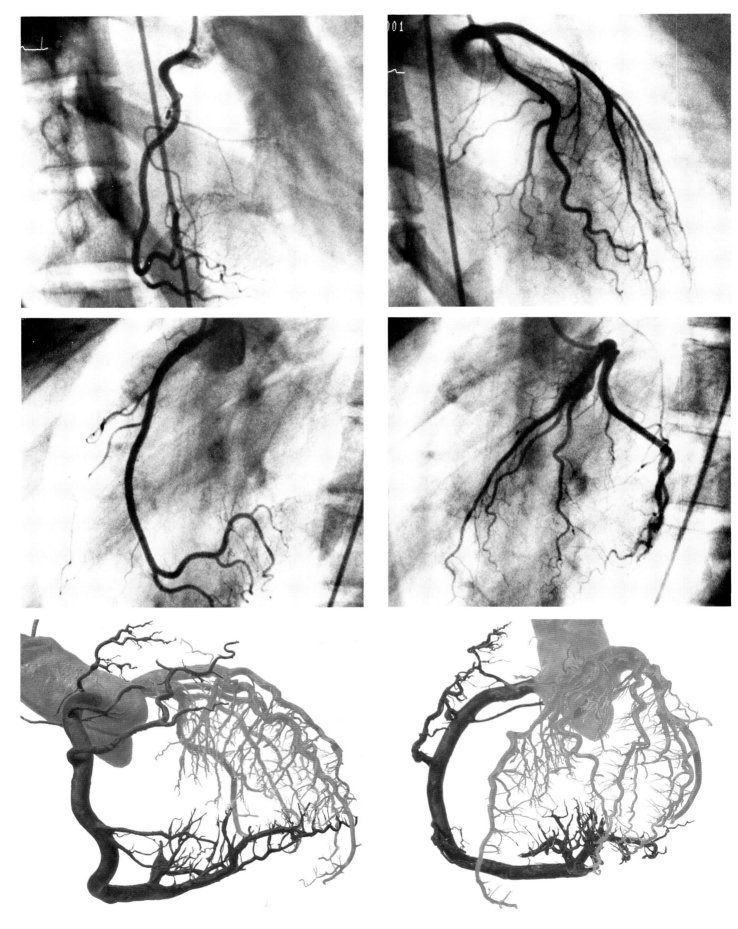

FIG. 47 Arteriograms of the right coronary artery. Top: right anterior oblique aspect; middle, left anterior oblique aspect; bottom: resin specimen (right anterior oblique view). (Resin specimen courtesy Dr. Kumiko Tanuma, Department of Anatomy, Nippon Medical School.)

FIG. 48 Arteriograms of the left coronary artery. Top: right anterior oblique aspect; middle: left anterior oblique aspect; bottom: resin specimen (left anterior oblique aspect). (Resin specimen courtesy Dr. Kumiko Tanuma, Department of Anatomy, Nippon Medical School.)

Pathologic Examination

POSTMORTEM CORONARY ANGIOGRAPHY

Postmortem coronary angiography is useful in determining the sites of coronary artery lesions before their pathologic examination. Whenever possible, coronary artery angiography should be performed, exercising caution to avoid arterial damage that may interfere with pathologic examination.

A commercially available box-type soft x-ray camera is suitable for postmortem angiography. This camera is easy to use and does not require x-ray exposure testing or application for use in a designated area. However, one disadvantage is high cost, and ordinary x-ray equipment may be used instead. The radiographic conditions can be the same as those used for soft x-ray examination of the breast. For x-ray film, compact Kodak A4 size film is commercially available.

Generally, the contrast medium is prepared by combining 100 g of barium with 100 ml of water and heating to 45°C. Gelatin (5 g) is then added and dissolved. If urgency prevails, the barium preparation used for gastric fluoroscopy can be used, but it is necessary to thoroughly wash away the barium after angiography to avoid adverse effects on the pathologic examination.

The proximal aspects of the left and right coronary arteries are exposed, and a cannula is introduced into each artery. The cannulae are then tightly secured with silk sutures, applied near the origin of each artery to prevent dislodgment. Blood remaining in the vessels is judiciously and thoroughly removed by washing the arteries with physiologic saline. The vessels are then filled with physiologic saline using a three-way stopcock,

and slowly injected with the barium preparation at a pressure of 100 to 200 mmHg. Preliminary angiography should then be attempted two or three times to evaluate the injected dose of barium. Arteriography is usually initiated from the healthy vessels, and if the contralateral vessels are visualized through the collateral circulation, they do not have to undergo arteriography separately. Care is required not to dislodge any occlusive thrombi or damage the stenotic lesions at the orifice. Figure 49 presents an example of postmortem coronary angiography.

HISTOLOGIC EXAMINATION

The intrapericardial coronary arteries are dissected from the heart after adequate fixation. Decalcification is performed if required. The left main trunk, right coronary, left anterior descending, and left circumflex arteries are then transversely sectioned at intervals of 3 to 5 mm. After macroscopic inspection, the sections are photographed and arranged into a complete coronary artery specimen (Fig. 50). The sections are then dehydrated, embedded in paraffin, prepared into thinly sliced and intact specimens, and stained with hematoxylin-eosin (HE), Masson trichrome, elastica van Gieson, or PTAH stain. Serial sections are prepared if necessary.

The degree of stenosis caused by atherosclerotic plaques of the coronary arteries is generally calculated by the following formula, designating the patent lumen to be oval-shaped.

$$\text{Degree of stenosis} = \frac{0.25 \times p \times D \times d}{pr^2 \times 100}$$

where D = longest diameter; d = shortest diameter; r = radius, designating the internal elastic lamina to be circular.

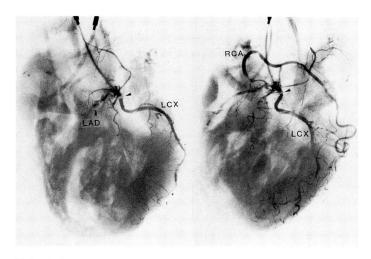

FIG. 49 Postmortem coronary arteriography. (LAD, left anterior oblique aspect; LCX, left circumflex artery; RCA, right coronary artery.)

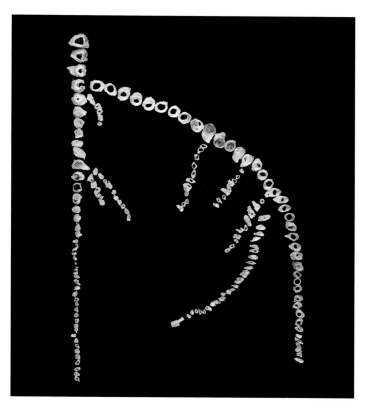

FIG. 50 Examination method of coronary arteries. The left coronary artery was sectioned transversely at intervals of 3 to 5 mm and examined.

3. Angina Pectoris

Angina pectoris is a syndrome characterized mainly by episodes of chest pain arising from myocardial ischemia. Although the mechanism responsible for intermittent chest pain has not been fully defined, the most convincing theory ascribes this phenomenon to anaerobic metabolism in the myocardium.

Myocardial ischemia is caused by disruption of the oxygen demand-supply equilibrium of the myocardium. More specifically, myocardial ischemia may result when (1) increases in coronary blood flow cannot meet increased oxygen consumption by the myocardium, (2) the coronary blood flow transiently declines, or (3) a combination of these factors. Classic effort angina is caused by the former mechanism. Specifically, when the effort-induced increase in myocardial oxygen demand attains a certain level, it can no longer be met by the rise in blood flow restricted by stenotic lesions associated with coronary arteriosclerosis, thus leading to the breakdown of the myocardial oxygen supply-demand equilibrium. Initially, myocardial ischemia occurs on the endocardial side, with its higher intramyocardial pressure, and chest pains appear. The degree of stenosis at which coronary blood flow cannot meet demand is estimated to be ≥90% of the cross-sectional area of the coronary artery during rest or ≥75% during exercise (Fig. 60). The greater the severity of the stenosis and the greater the number of stenotic vessels, the lower the threshold for the onset of myocardial ischemia. In effort angina pectoris with severe organic stenotic lesions, myocardial ischemia may be caused by even a slight increase in myocardial oxygen demand, such as that produced by emotional stress.

If basic oxygen demand in effort angina pectoris is elevated because of associated conditions such as hyperthyroidism or anemia, the threshold of myocardial oxygen imbalance is lowered.

In angina pectoris caused by coronary spasm, by contrast, the epicardially situated coronary artery main trunk is occluded during an attack, transiently interrupting coronary blood flow. Consequently, transmural myocardial ischemia occurs in association with attacks of chest pain (Fig. 59). If spasm-induced occlusion of the coronary arteries is incomplete, myocardial ischemia may be localized on the endocardial side.

Recently, coronary angiography has been actively carried out during the acute phase of unstable angina pectoris. Such studies have detected a high prevalence of occlusive thrombi, and anginal attacks have been alleviated by intracoronary injection of thrombolytic agents (Fig. 61). Therefore, thrombi also appear to be important in the mechanism of myocardial ischemia, as well as organic stenosis and spasm.

The most expedient and useful method for diagnosing angina pectoris is recording electrocardiographic (ECG) changes during an attack. Diagnosis can be confirmed on the basis of occurrence of ST segment depression or elevation, during an attack, on standard 12-lead ECG, or long-term ECG (Fig. 51). If a spontaneous attack cannot be recorded, episodes of angina may be induced by exercise tests or by the induction of coronary spasm in hyperventilation tests, cold pressor tests, or the administration of drugs such as ergonovine. The most sensitive examination currently used to diagnose the presence of ischemia is exercise myocardial scintigraphy (Figs. 52 to 55). By this method, the ischemic sites appear as thallium redistribution images.

In echocardiography, reduced left ventricular motility is noted during attacks (Figs. 56 to 58).

Table 1 shows three standard classifications of angina pectoris.

Table 1. Classification of Angina Pectoris

ISFC/WHO classification	AHA classification
1. Angina pectoris on effort: Characterized by transient attacks of chest pain induced by conditions such as exercise, which lead to increased myocardial oxygen demand. The chest pain is usually rapidly alleviated by rest or sublingual administration of nitroglycerin. Angina pectoris on effort is classified into the following three types: A. New angina pectoris on effort: Less than 1 month after onset B. Stable angina pectoris on effort: Duration of 1 month or longer C. Unstable or aggravated angina pectoris on effort: The frequency, intensity, and duration of chest pain caused by the same effort suddenly become worse 2. Angina pectoris at rest: Characterized by attacks of chest pain that appear with no definite relation to increased myocardial oxygen demand. Chest pains last longer and are more severe than in effort angina pectoris, and the effect of nitroglycerin tends to be delayed.	Cases where chest pain as indicated below starts within 3 weeks before hospitalization, with the last episode of chest pain occurring within 1 week. No ECG findings of new myocardial infarctions or elevation of myocardial enzymes is evident. 1. New angina pectoris on effort: New occurrence of chest pains during effort or recurrence after an asymptomatic period of at least 6 months. 2. Aggravated angina pectoris on effort: Previously stable angina pectoris on effort, which shows increases in the frequency, intensity, and duration of chest pain attacks. The efficacy of sublingual nitroglycerin frequently declines. 3. New angina pectoris at rest: Attacks of chest pain occur at rest. Attacks occasionally persisting for more than 15 minutes are not always alleviated by nitroglycerin. Transient ST segment changes (elevation or depression) or T-wave inversion is often seen in the ECG during chest pain.

Other types of angina pectoris	
1. Variant angina pectoris (Am J Med 27:375, 1959): Prinzmetal proposed that a form of angina pectoris characterized by pain only at rest and ST segment elevation during an attack be called variant angina pectoris. It most often appears at night or in the early morning. The mechanism of variant angina has been shown to be coronary spasm. 2. Coronary spasm angina pectoris: Refers to angina pectoris caused by the transient occurrence of complete or semicomplete functional occlusion of the coronary arteries (coronary spasm without severe organic stenosis). Attacks occur mainly at rest and show ST seg-	ment elevation, while attacks precipitated by exercise show remarkable variations in their induction threshold. Calcium antagonists are often effective. 3. Postinfarction angina pectoris: Angina pectoris that occurs during the period from 24 hours after acute myocardial infarction until discharge. May be caused by ischemia of viable myocardium remaining in the infarcted area or its periphery, or by severe stenosis of vessels supplying noninfarcted areas.

FIG. 51 Exercise ECGs in effort angina pectoris (90% stenosis of left anterior descending artery). ST segment depression can be seen in leads V$_{3-6}$ during exercise.

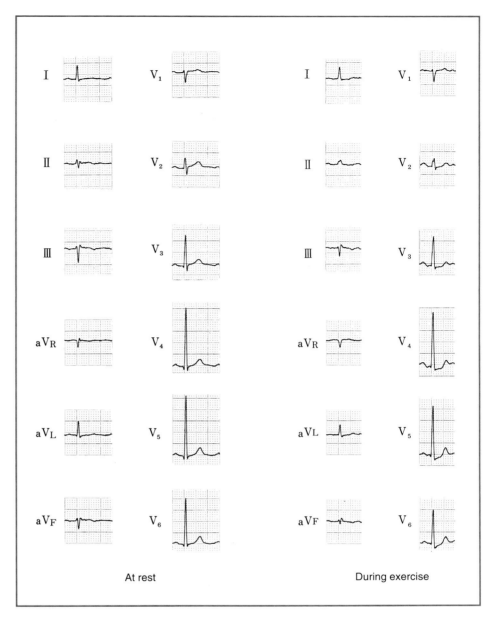

FIG. 52 Exercise myocardial scintigrams (planar images) in effort angina pectoris (90% stenosis of left anterior descending artery). a: frontal surface; b: left anterior oblique 40° aspect; c: left anterior oblique 70° aspect. Defect regions, evident in the anterior septum during exercise (EX), disappear during redistribution (RD).

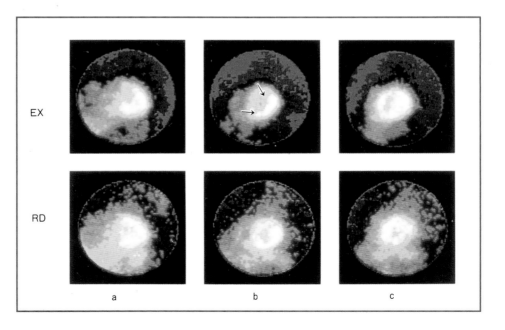

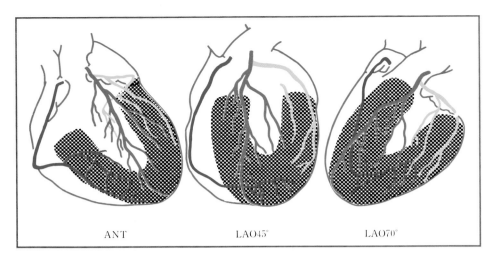

FIG. 53 Regions supplied by the coronary arteries in myocardial planar images. The red, yellow, and blue lines indicate the left anterior descending artery, left circumflex artery, and right coronary artery, respectively.

ANT   LAO45°   LAO70°

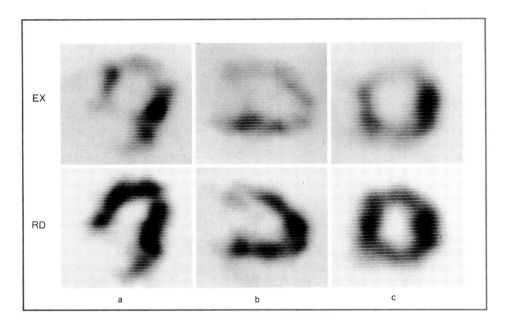

FIG. 54 Exercise myocardial scintigrams (SPECT images) in effort angina pectoris. a: body axis CT image; b: long-axis CT image; c: short-axis CT image. Defect areas corresponding to the anterior wall can be seen during exercise (EX), but disappear on redistribution (RD).

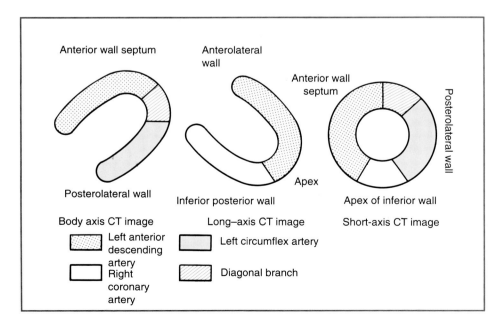

FIG. 55 Myocardial region classification and the corresponding dominant coronary arteries by myocardial SPECT.

FIG. 56 Long-axis cardiac echograms during anginal attack. a,b: no attack; c,d: during anginal attack; a,c: diastole; b,d: systole. Reduced motility of the interventricular septum is evident in d.

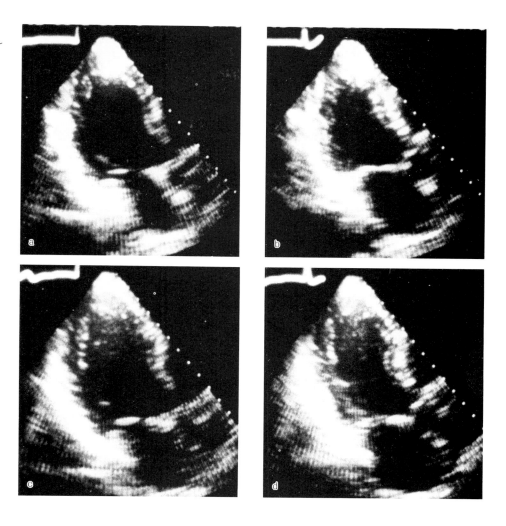

FIG. 57 Short-axis cardiac echograms during anginal attack in the same patient as shown in Fig. 56. a,b: no attack; c,d: during anginal attack; a,c: diastole; b,d: systole. Contraction of the anterior wall septum is not evident (d).

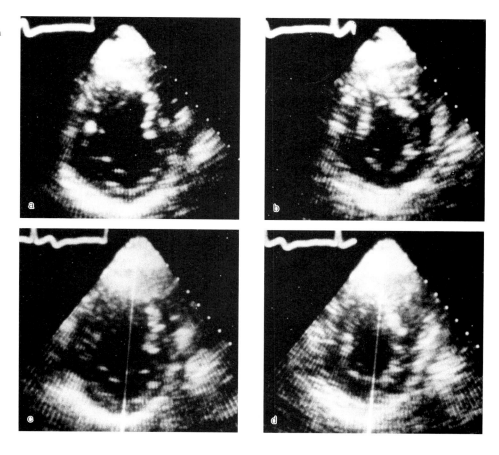

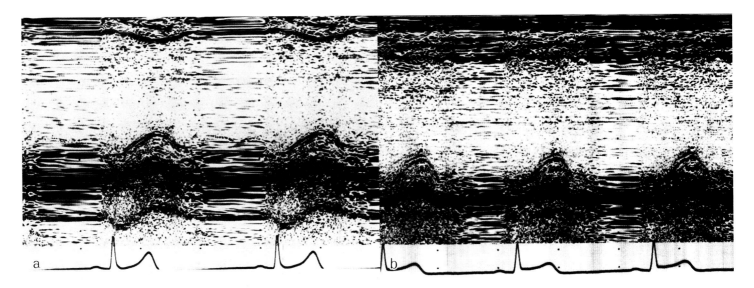

FIG. 58 M-mode echocardiogram during anginal attack in the patient shown in Fig. 56. a: normal control; b: during anginal attack. During an attack, inward movement of the septum disappears.

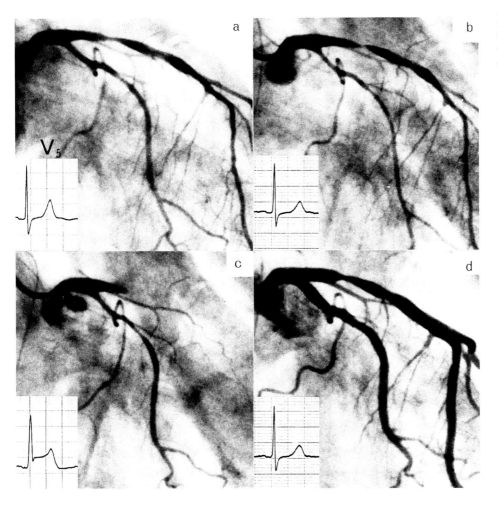

FIG. 59 Coronary angiograms. Coronary spasms. a: normal control; b: hyperventilation; c: intracoronary injection of ergonovine; d: intracoronary injection of TNG.

Pathologic Aspects

GROSS FINDINGS

When myocardial necrosis occurs in the region supplied by the coronary arteries, and the longest diameter of the outer border of the myocardial necrosis exceeds 1 cm, the lesion is generally defined as a myocardial infarct.

Myocardial infarctions are classified as being transmural or subendocardial. The former extends beyond half the ventricular wall thickness, and the latter, involving less than half of the ventricular wall thickness, remains on the endocardial side. At autopsy, the heart is weighed and its surface is examined (for fibrosis, pericarditis, etc.). Usually without sectioning, blood is removed from the cardiac lumen, and the heart is fixed in 10% neutral buffered formalin. After sufficient fixation (3 to 7 days), horizontal sections are prepared at approximately 1 cm intervals from the apex of the heart and observed (Fig. 78). The transverse sections, including the maximum area of the infarction, and sections showing other specific findings are embedded in paraffin, large tissue specimens about 5 mm thick are prepared, and the area of the infarction is examined (Fig. 79). Staining methods used include HE stain, Masson trichrome, elastica van Gieson, PTAH, and Heidenhain's iron hematoxylin stain.

The infarcted area can be readily quantified by calculating the infarcted area relative to the total ventricular transverse area in the large tissue specimens using a personal computer.

In addition, methods for macroscopic diagnosis of myocardial infarctions include identifying the infarcted area by staining the nonfixed myocardium with nitro-blue tetrazolium (NBT) or triphenyl tetrazolium chloride (TTC). Both stains possess high affinities for dehydrogenase, which is released from the necrotic area. This method enables detection of necrotic areas 4 hours after the onset of infarction, making it useful for the diagnosis of early infarctions.

In the generally used TTC method, TTC reagent is first dissolved in 0.2 M TRIS buffer (pH 8.0–8.5) and then heated to 37°C to prepare a 1% solution. The nonfixed myocardium is cut into sections less than 1 cm thick, allowed to stand in the solution for 1 hour at 37° to 40°C, and then refrigerated overnight at 4°C. Normal myocardium reacts with TTC and turns a dark red color because of the presence of dehydrogenase succinate, whereas no color change occurs with ischemic myocardium because the enzyme has already escaped (Fig. 80).

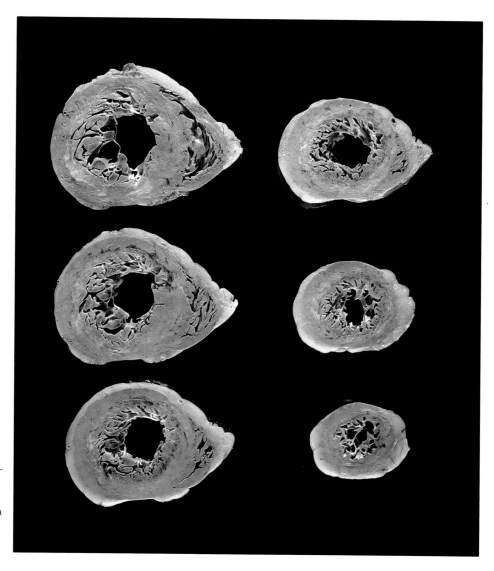

FIG. 78 Myocardial infarction examination method. After fixing the heart in formalin, horizontal sections are cut at intervals of about 1 cm, starting at the apex, and examined. An old myocardial infarction appears to be white, and a myocardial infarction that occurred about 2 weeks previously is blackish brown.

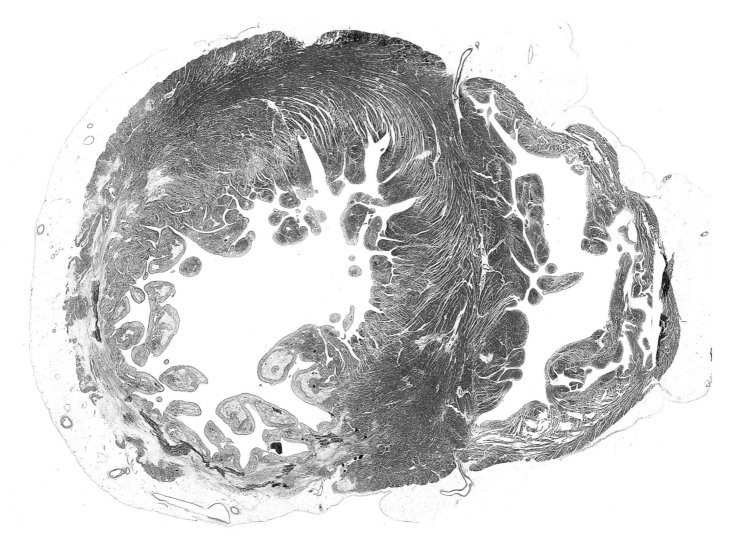

FIG. 79 Histologic transverse section. A myocardial infarction consisting of a fibrous area stained light blue and a necrotic coagulation
area stained reddish violet were noted in the posterolateral wall of the
left ventricle. (Masson trichrome stain.)

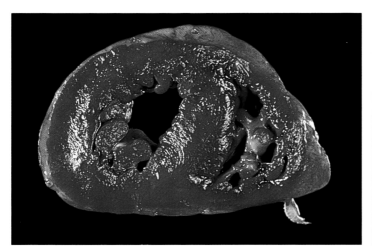 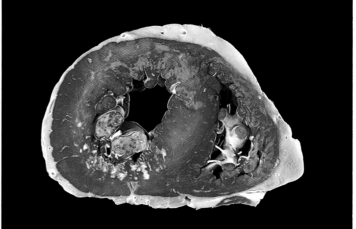

FIG. 80 TTC treatment (before and after). In this transverse section
before TTC treatment (left figure), only a whitish fibrous area is seen
in the posterior wall of the left ventricle. After TTC treatment (right
figure), the healthy myocardium is stained red. A yellowish-brown
unstained region is present in the anterior wall of the left ventricle,
indicating a myocardial infarct. The fibrous area in the posterior wall,
also not stained, has a whitish color. Most of the right ventricular wall
is unstained, but this is unrelated to a myocardial infarction. The evaluation of infarction of the right ventricle is difficult with this method.

DATING OF MYOCARDIAL INFARCTIONS Mallory et al. (1939) and Loge-Patch (1951) published detailed reports on serial changes in the myocardium after the onset of infarction. These reports are still often quoted in reference to the time course of infarcted tissue. Briefly, it is difficult to determine macroscopically whether an infarction is present 5 to 6 hours after onset. On palpation of a cross-section of the infarction, it feels somewhat soft and its color bears a light red hue. However, the initial findings in infarction are visible at this stage by light microscopy. First, coagulation necrosis of the myocardial fibers is evident. The cell bodies show increased eosinophilic staining, and the striations have disappeared. The nuclei are darkly stained or are no longer evident.

Infarctions are most easily distinguished macroscopically about 2 to 3 days after onset. The infarcted area becomes very soft, and the color changes from reddish brown to even pink, depending on the degree of cellular infiltration. Histologically, interstitial edema increases, and marked infiltration of neutrophils proceeds from the margin to the center of the infarction.

Thinning of the infarcted area occurs 4 to 7 days after onset. Because the infarcted area undergoes granulation, whitish tissue surrounding the brownish central region forms a distinct boundary with the noninfarcted myocardium. Especially dramatic at the margin of the infarction, liquefaction and absorption of the necrotic myocardium are evident; neutrophils start to decrease in the interstices and are replaced by lymphocytes, macrophages, and fibroblasts. Capillaries also proliferate.

By 12 to 14 days after infarction, the proliferation of young collagen fibers can be seen among fibroblasts and macrophages. Macroscopically, the whitish color also becomes more prominent. About 2 months after infarction, cellular components diminish and are replaced by dense collagen fibers. Macroscopically, a distinct whitish tone appears and tightly fibrous cicatricial foci are formed. Six months after infarction, no appreciable cellular components remain; fibrosis is complete and gelatinization occurs.

Histologic changes after myocardial infarction generally follow this typical healing process. However, large infarctions, infarctions associated with chronic ischemia, and hemorrhagic infarctions may present with slight variations in the healing process. Large infarctions take longer to heal than small infarctions of 1 to 2 cm, and coagulation necrosis of the myocardium may remain for a prolonged period in the center of the infarction.

When an infarction occurs in the presence of chronic ischemia, both new and old necrotic foci may be present histologically; as often occurs in subendocardial infarction, the healing mechanism may not proceed normally even after coagulation necrosis develops, and the neutrophil response is frequently poor. In such instances, dating the myocardial infarction from histologic findings is difficult. The repair process is often similarly prolonged in hemorrhagic infarction (Fig. 97).

HISTOLOGY OF EARLY MYOCARDIAL INFARCTION Infarction foci within 6 hours of onset generally show few histologic changes visible by light microscopy, and the definitive identification of an infarction is often deceptive. In such cases, infarction is frequently diagnosed by referring to clinical findings and coronary artery lesions detected by postmortem angiography, based on corresponding findings such as wavy changes to myocardial fibers, interstitial edema, margination by intracapillary neutrophils, and eosinophilic changes of cell bodies and karyopyknosis in myocardial fibers.

In early myocardial infarction, contraction band necrosis is often found. It is apparently triggered by reperfusion disturbances, but the details are unclear. Morphologically, the myocardial cells are in a state of overcontraction, and highly eosinophilic contraction bands appear (Fig. 99).

Recently, immunoenzyme antibody techniques have been used to identify early myocardial infarctions by staining myocardial proteins such as myoglobin and myosin, but this procedure is not widely used.

Minute changes in the myocardium in early infarction can be observed by electron microscopy, which is useful in diagnosis. However, this method is expensive, requires a long time for examination, and is difficult with respect to determining the extent of the infarction.

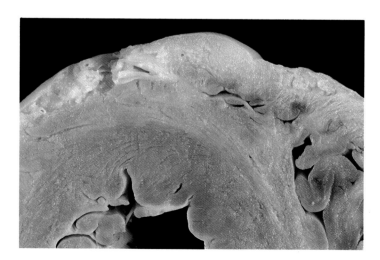

FIG. 81 Sequential changes (6 hours). About one-half of the endocardial side of the myocardium is a dark brown color, the muscle bundles have separated due to edema, and gaps can be seen.

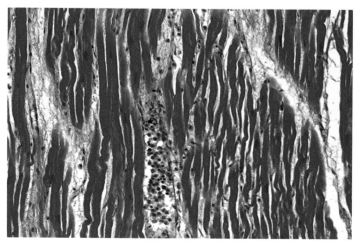

FIG. 82 Sequential changes (6 hours). The myocardial fibers show strong eosinophilic staining, and karyopyknosis is evident. Interstitial edema and neutrophilic margination of the capillaries can be noted. (HE stain, × 130.)

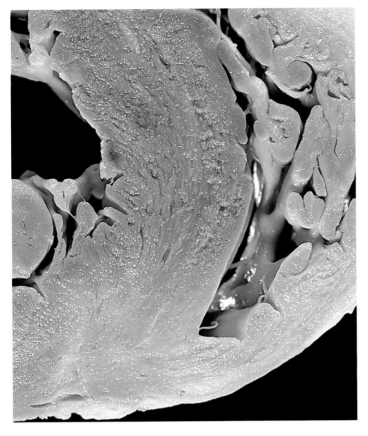

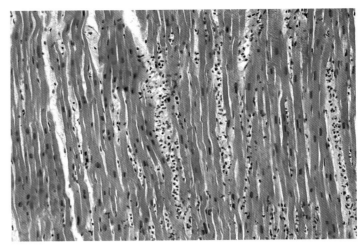

FIG. 84 Sequential changes (16 hours). Myocardial cells show eosinophilic staining and wavy changes. The striations have disappeared, and karyopyknosis and interstitial neutrophil infiltration are evident. (HE stain, × 130.)

FIG. 83 Sequential changes (16 hours). Most of the intraventricular septum is dark brown and the surface is rough because of interstitial edema.

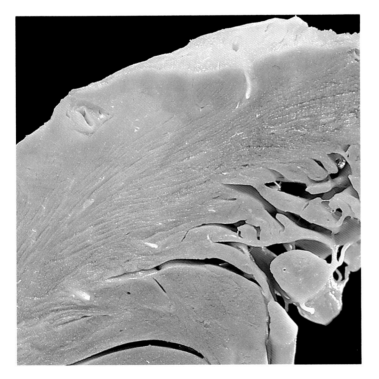

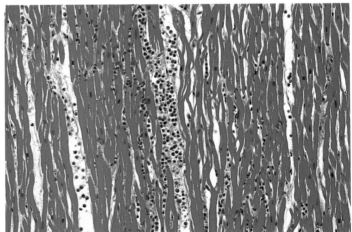

FIG. 86 Sequential changes (31 hours). The myocardial fibers show strong eosinophilic staining, striations have disappeared, and karyopyknosis and denucleation are observed. Marked neutrophil infiltration can be seen interstitially. (HE stain, × 130.)

FIG. 85 Sequential changes (31 hours). The anterior wall of the left ventricle has changed to a blackish brown color and mild thinning is seen. Surface roughness is also evident.

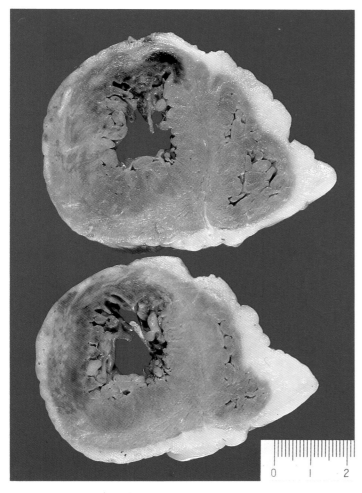

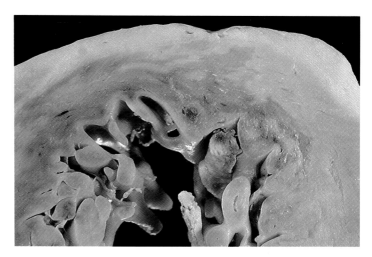

FIG. 108 Magnification of the infarction focus. Slightly white, transparent granulation tissue is intermingled with the surviving myocardium around the infarcted region. Coagulation necrosis, brownish in color with a small area of hemorrhage, is principally evident subendocardially.

FIG. 107 Transverse sections. Level about one-third from the apex. Transmural discoloration with bleeding can be seen in the anterolateral wall of the left ventricle. The anterior wall is rather thin, and the ventricular cavity is enlarged.

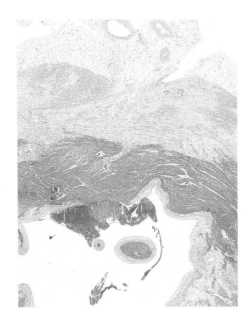

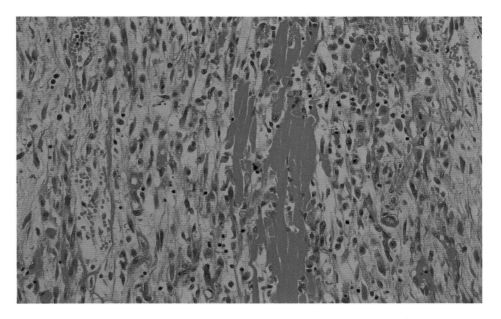

FIG. 110 Histologic findings in the anterior wall of the left ventricle. Granulation changes are present epicardially, and some surviving myocardium is also evident. Coagulation necrosis persists subendocardially, and mural thrombi can be noted. (Masson trichrome stain, × 5.5.)

FIG. 111 Histologic findings in the infarcted area. Coagulation necrosis of the myocardium and signs of the repair process are seen. Infiltration of histocytes, small round cells, and fibroblasts can be seen together with small hemorrhage sites. Almost no neutrophils are present. (HE stain, × 130.)

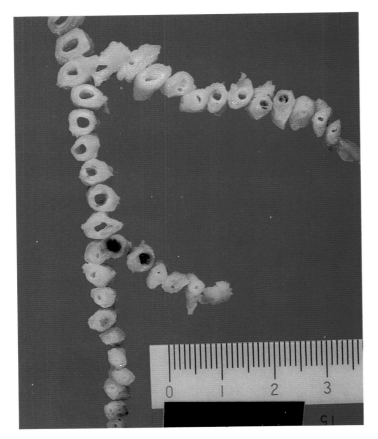

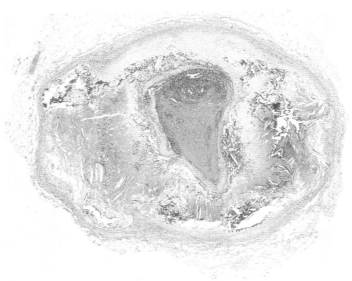

FIG. 113 First diagonal branch of the left coronary artery. The lumen is narrowed by an atheroma, and complete occlusion by a thrombus can be seen. (Masson trichrome stain, × 18.5.)

FIG. 112 Left coronary artery. The first diagonal branch just after bifurcation is completely occluded with hemorrhage in the atheroma. More than 75% stenosis is seen in the left anterior descending artery (segment 7) and the left circumflex artery.

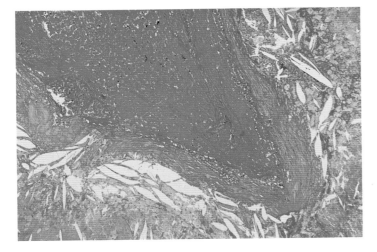

FIG. 114 First diagonal branch of the left coronary artery. Rupture of the atheroma and thrombi can be noted. The fibrin net of the thrombi is darkly stained and presents with a uniform appearance. (HE stain, × 65.)

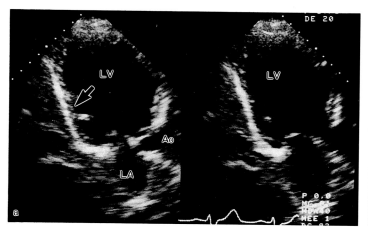
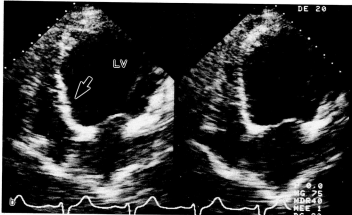

FIG. 165 Echocardiograms. a: the thickness of the posterior wall has decreased (arrow) and increased brightness is seen. b: reduced wall thickness (arrow) and decreased motility are evident in the septum. (Ao, aorta; LA, left atrium; LV, left ventricle.)

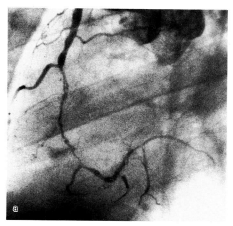
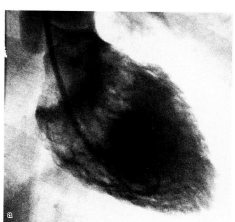
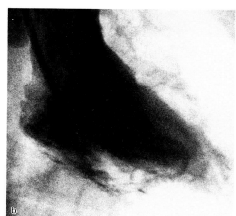

FIG. 167 Left ventriculography. a: end-diastole; b: end-systole.

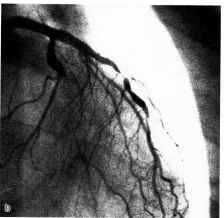

FIG. 166 Coronary angiography. a: right coronary artery; b: left coronary artery.

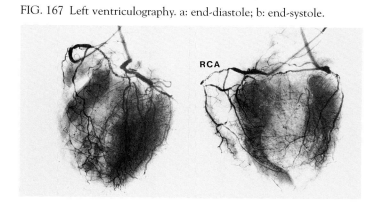

FIG. 168 Postmortem angiography. (RCA, right coronary artery.)

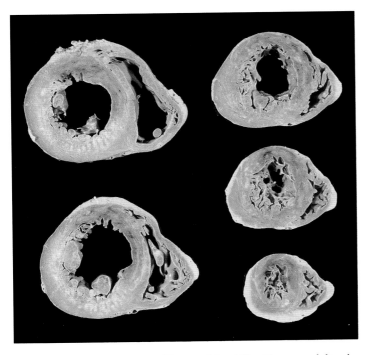

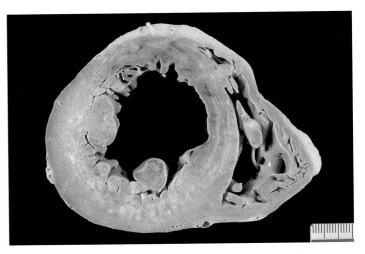

FIG. 170 Transverse section. Level of the center of the papillary muscles. Areas of discoloration are noted in the anterior portion of the interventricular septum and anterior wall of the left ventricle. In the posterolateral wall, an old infarction, which is mainly subendocardial but partially transmural, can be seen. Fibrosis and discoloration are also evident in the papillary muscles. Slight thinning can be observed in the anterior part of the septum and the anterior wall.

FIG. 169 Transverse sections. Heart weight: 450 g. Transmural discolored areas can be seen in the anterior portion of the interventricular septum and anterior wall of the left ventricle from the base of the heart to the apex. An old transmural myocardial infarction, whitish in color, is evident in the posterior wall of the left ventricle. The left ventricular cavity is enlarged.

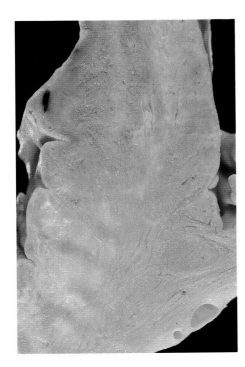

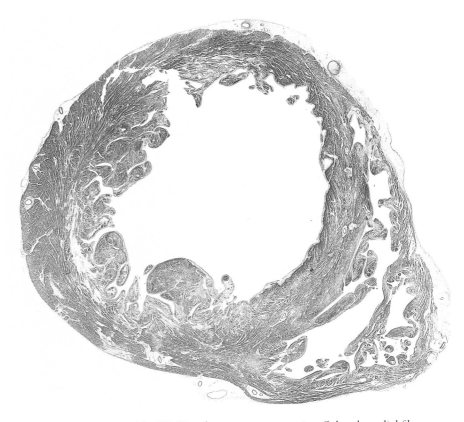

FIG. 171 Close-up view of the infarction area. The anterior portion of the interventricular septum is discolored and slightly indented. The paths of the myocardial fibers are difficult to follow and the surface is rough. The boundary with the normal myocardium is distinct. Slightly transparent white fibrous areas intermingle with viable myocardium in the posterior wall of the left ventricle.

FIG. 172 Histologic transverse section. Subendocardial fibrous areas are mainly evident in the posterior wall of the left ventricle. In the anterior portion of the interventricular septum and the anterior wall of the left ventricle, myocardial fibers are wavy and show reduced stainability. (Masson trichrome stain.)

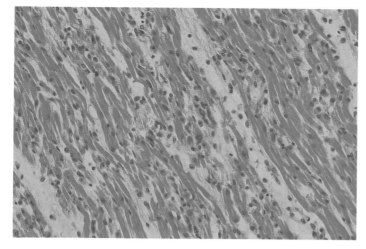

FIG. 173 Histologic findings in the infarction in the anterior wall of the left ventricle. The myocardial fibers show eosinophilic staining and are thin, wavy, and ruptured. The striated structure and nuclei have disappeared. The interstices are edematous and the myocardial fibers are disaggregated. Neutrophil infiltration has declined and histocyte infiltration is evident. (HE stain, × 130.)

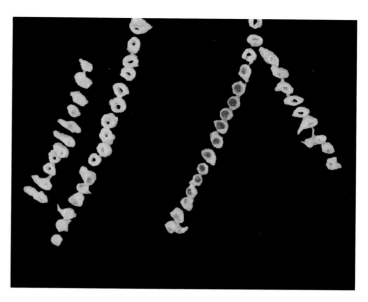

FIG. 174 Coronary arteries. The proximal portion (segment 6) of the left anterior descending artery shows atheromatous hemorrhage and complete occlusion caused by thrombosis. In the distal portion (segment 13) of the left circumflex artery and peripherally from the middle portion of the right coronary artery (segment 2 and 3), severe stenosis of more than 90% can be seen.

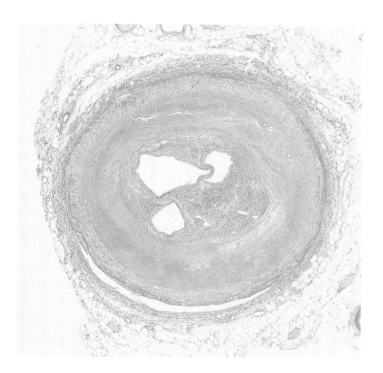

FIG. 175 Histologic findings in the right coronary artery. Recanalization is evident. (Masson trichrome stain, × 21.)

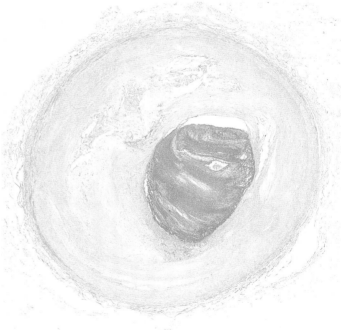

FIG. 176 Histologic findings in the left anterior descending artery. Complete occlusion by an atheroma and a laminated thrombus is evident. (Masson trichrome stain, × 17.5.)

Case 7 Inferior Wall Infarction (8 hours), Anterior Wall Infarction (3 years 8 months)

The patient was a 49-year-old man who smoked 30 cigarettes a day. He had no history of hypertension, but had diabetes mellitus. He was hospitalized locally for an anterior wall septal infarction 3 years and 8 months before death, and angina pectoris continued after the infarction. Eight months before death, left ventriculography and coronary angiography revealed complete occlusion of segment 6 of the left anterior descending artery; 75% stenosis of segment 13 of the left circumflex artery; no contraction of the anterolateral wall, apex, or septal wall; and reduced contraction of the diaphragmatic, posterobasal, and posterolateral walls. The cardiac index was 3.2 L/min/m² and the ejection fraction was 32%. One day before death, the patient complained of difficulty in breathing, which was alleviated by nitroglycerin, but he was hospitalized because of the persistence of frequent attacks. Dyspnea suddenly occurred 8 hours before death. ST segment elevation was seen in leads II, III, and $_aV_F$ on the ECG. An inferior wall infarction was diagnosed. The mean pulmonary wedge pressure was 6 mmHg and the cardiac index was 3.79 L/min/m². The patient was Killip I and Forrester I. Two hours before death, there was a shift from short runs of ventricular extrasystoles to ventricular tachycardia and ventricular fibrillation. The patient did not respond to drug treatment and died.

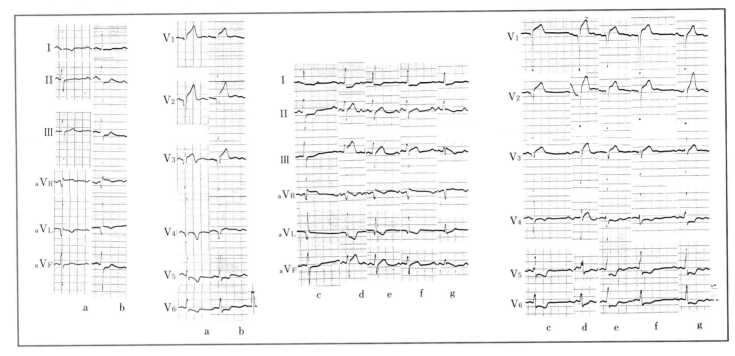

FIG. 177 Electrocardiograms. a: 1 year 8 months before onset of myocardial infarct; b–g: day of myocardial infarct; c: 07:16, d: 08:10, e: 08:50, f: 10:13, g: 12:20.

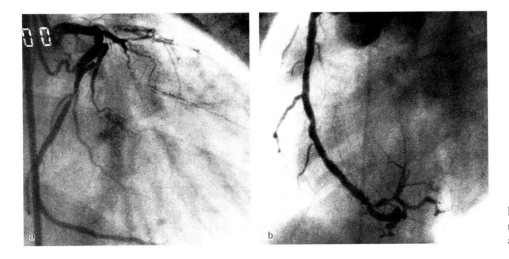

FIG. 178 Coronary angiography. a: left coronary artery before infarction; b: right coronary artery.

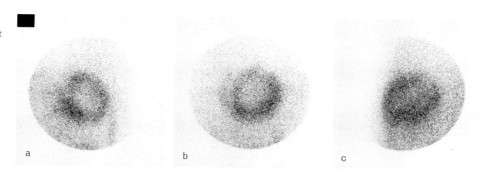

FIG. 179 Myocardial scintigrams. a: frontal aspect; b: left anterior oblique 45° aspect; c: left lateral aspect. Defect images are seen from the anterior wall to part of the inferior wall.

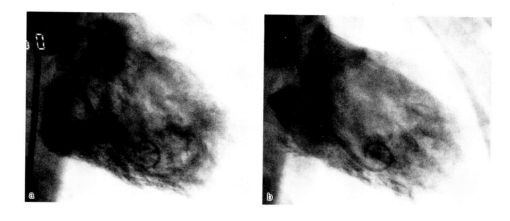

FIG. 180 Left ventriculography. a: end-diastole; b: end-systole.

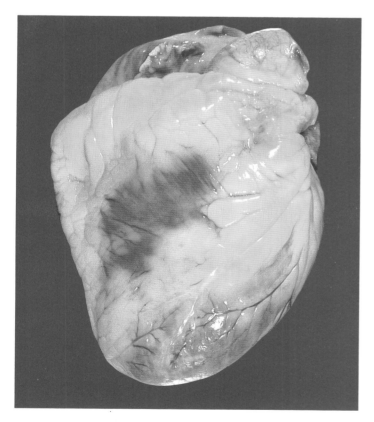

FIG. 181 Frontal surface of the heart. Heart weight: 470 g. The apex consists of the left ventricle. The epicardium of the anterior wall of the left ventricle and the apex is hypertrophied and white.

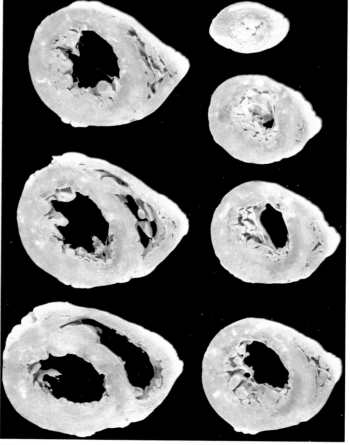

FIG. 182 Transverse sections. Fibrous areas are mainly situated subendocardially in the anterior portion of the interventricular septum and the anterolateral wall of the left ventricle from the base to the apex of the heart. Near the apex, the fibrosis is transmural. An area of discoloration from the posterior portion of the interventricular septum to the posterior wall is present, and the left ventricular cavity is enlarged.

Left Ventricular Infarction 85

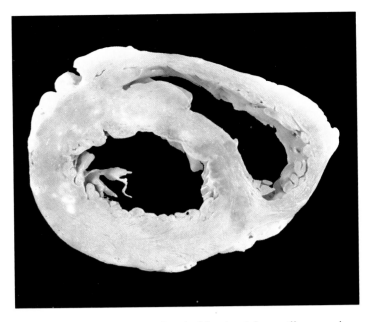

FIG. 183 Transverse section. Level of the tip of the papillary muscles. White subendocardial fibrous areas are seen in the anterior portion of the interventricular septum and the anterolateral wall of the left ventricle. An area of discoloration is present in the posterior portion of the interventricular septum.

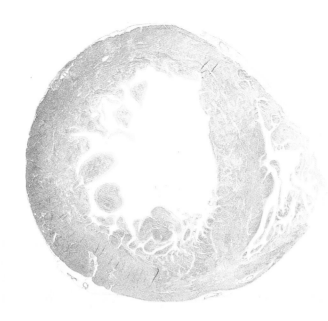

FIG. 184 Transverse histologic section. Fibrous areas are mainly present subendocardially in the anterior portion of the interventricular septum and the anterior wall of the left ventricle. Changes in staining properties are evident in part of the posterior portion of the interventricular septum and the posterior wall of the left ventricle.

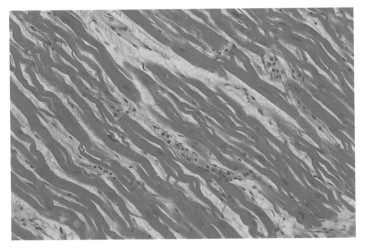

FIG. 185 Infarction area in the posterior portion of the interventricular septum. The myocardial fibers show eosinophilic staining. They are fine, wavy, and dissociated. The striated structure and nuclei are still present. The interstitium is edematous and neutrophil margination is evident. (HE stain, × 180.)

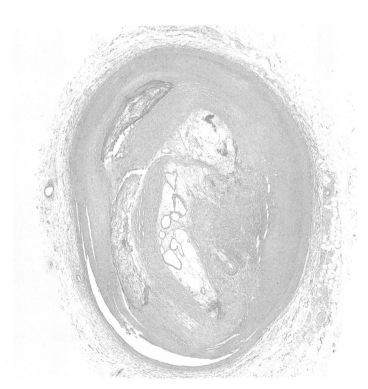

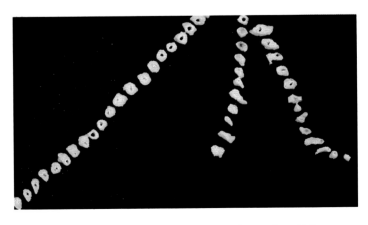

FIG. 186 Coronary arteries. Severe stenosis of more than 90% is seen in the right coronary artery (segment 2), left anterior descending artery (segment 6), and left circumflex artery (segment 13.)

FIG. 187 Histologic findings in the left anterior descending artery. Recanalization is evident. (Masson trichrome stain.)

CASE 8 SUBENDOCARDIAL INFARCTION (CONCENTRIC, 3 DAYS)

The patient was an 82-year-old man who smoked 10 to 40 cigarettes a day. He was hypertensive but not diabetic. Ten years before death, the patient became aware of shortness of breath on exertion. Three days before death severe dyspnea occurred at about 5 AM but symptoms were alleviated in about 30 minutes. At about 2 AM on the following day, breathing difficulty recurred and continued until morning. He was hospitalized at 4:30 PM. On admission his blood pressure was 124/80 mmHg and pulse was 140 beats/min and regular. He had orthopnea and rales were heard in both lung fields. The CK was 1,404 IU/L and the SGOT was 94 IU/L. On ECG elevation and depression of R waves were noted in leads V_{1-3} and ST segment depression was seen in leads I, II, $_aV_L$, and V_{2-6}. Blood pressure on admission dropped to 68 mmHg. The mean pulmonary artery wedge pressure was 20 mmHg, and the cardiac index was 2.09 L/min/m². Hemodynamics were stabilized by administration of positive inotropic agents and nitroglycerin, but 1 hour and 30 minutes before death ventricular tachycardia appeared. He did not respond to treatment and died. The maximum serum CK was 4,404 IU/L.

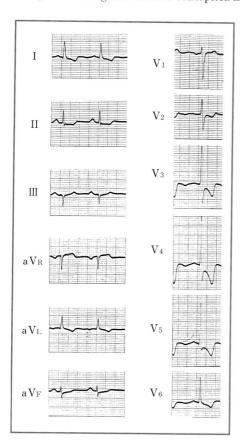

FIG. 188 Electrocardiograms. Day of infarction.

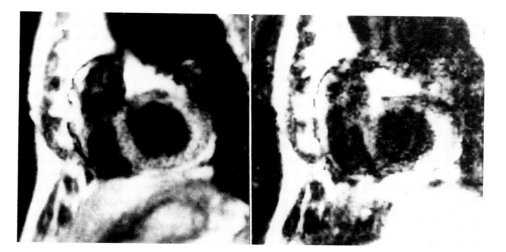

FIG. 189 ECG-synchronized MRI. Short-axis tomogram. A high-intensity area corresponding to the endocardial side is seen.

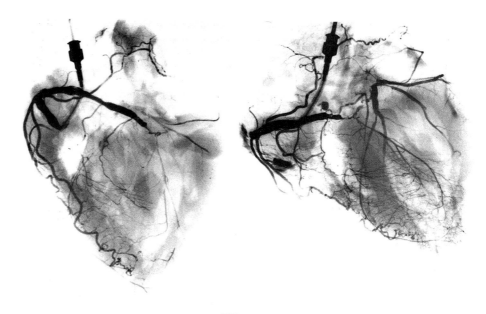

FIG. 190 Postmortem angiography.

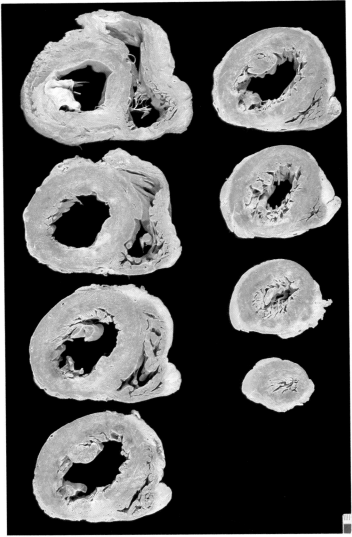

FIG. 191 Transverse sections. Heart weight: 485 g. Subendocardial discoloration extending throughout almost the entire circumference can be seen from the level of the tip end of the papillary muscles to the apex. White fibrous areas are also present. The ventricular cavity is enlarged.

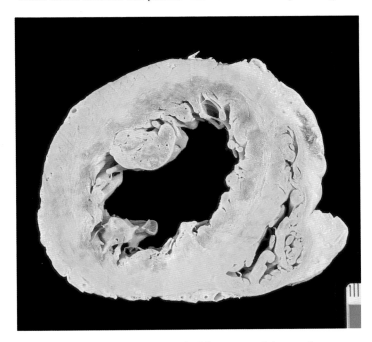

FIG. 192 Transverse section. Level of the center of the papillary muscles. Subendocardial discoloration is evident throughout the circumference of the left ventricle.

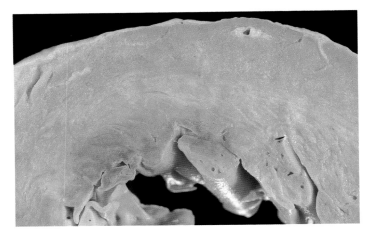

FIG. 193 Close-up view of the infarction focus. The discolored area with transparent white fibrous areas does not extend beyond half of the left ventricular muscle layer.

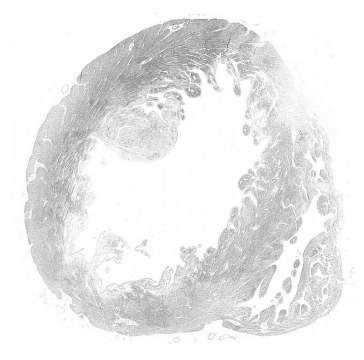

FIG. 194 Histologic transverse section. Blue fibrous areas are present in the papillary muscles and subendocardially throughout the circumference of the left ventricle. Areas stained a darker red than other regions are seen lining the areas of fibrosis. (Masson trichrome stain.)

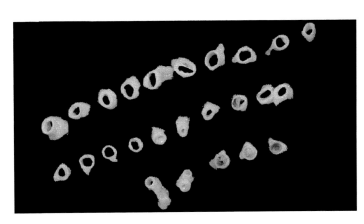

FIG. 197 Right coronary artery. Severe stenosis caused by an atheroma is evident in segment 3.

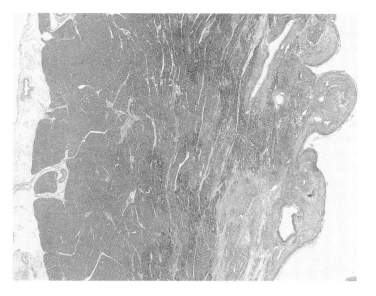

FIG. 195 Histologic findings in the lateral wall of the left ventricle. Old fibrous foci can be noted subendocardially and in the papillary muscles. The outer myocardial layer shows a wavy appearance and dark red staining. (Masson trichrome stain, × 8.)

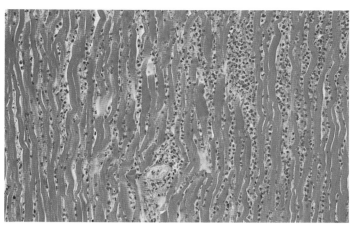

FIG. 196 Histologic findings. The myocardial cells are eosinophilic, the striations have disappeared, and denucleation has taken place. Marked inflammatory cell infiltration, consisting primarily of neutrophils, is evident. (HE stain, × 130.)

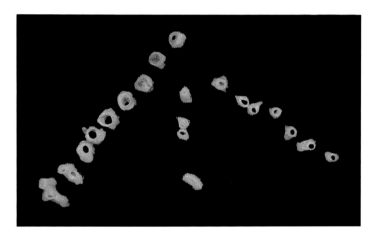

FIG. 199 Left coronary artery. Complete occlusion of the left anterior descending artery (segment 6) is seen.

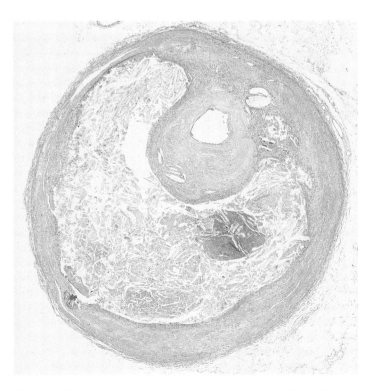

FIG. 198 Histologic findings in the distal part (segment 3) of the right coronary artery. (Masson trichrome stain, × 17.)

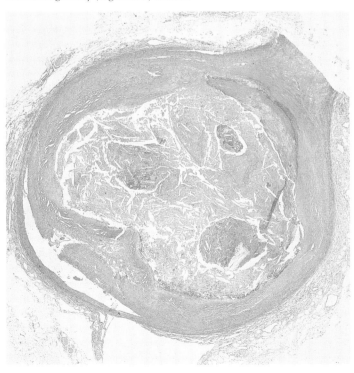

FIG. 200 Histologic findings in the proximal part (segment 6) of the left anterior descending artery. (Masson trichrome stain, × 14.5.)

CASE 9 SUBENDOCARDIAL INFARCTION (CONCENTRIC, 31 DAYS)

The patient was a 67-year-old man who was not hypertensive but had diabetes mellitus. Over the past 20 years, he occasionally experienced chest pains on exertion. For the past 4 years, frequent anginal pains had occurred. One year and 10 months before he was hospitalized for unstable angina pectoris and diabetes mellitus. Left ventriculography and coronary angiography revealed 90% stenosis of segment 1 of the right coronary artery, 90% stenosis of segment 6 of the left anterior descending artery, 75% stenosis of segment 11 and complete occlusion of segment 13 of the left circumflex artery, abnormal contraction of the anterolateral wall, no contraction of the apex or septal wall, and weakened contraction of the diaphragmatic wall.

The ejection fraction was 38%. The patient refused coronary artery bypass surgery and was discharged. Thereafter, anginal attacks and dyspnea ensued. Thirty-one days before death, persistent chest pain and orthopnea occurred from around 3 AM and he was admitted to the CCU at 10 AM. On admission, the blood pressure was 98/64 mmHg and the pulse rate 84 beats/min and regular. Rales were heard in both lung fields. The mean pulmonary artery wedge pressure was 33 mmHg, and the cardiac index was 1.92 L/min/m². The patient was classified as Killip IV and Forrester IV. An IABP was inserted to control heart failure. It was removed 2 days before the patient's death. One day before death, dyspnea appeared and the patient developed a low heart output syndrome and died. Maximum CK activity was 3,216 IU/L and maximum SGOT was 538 IU/L.

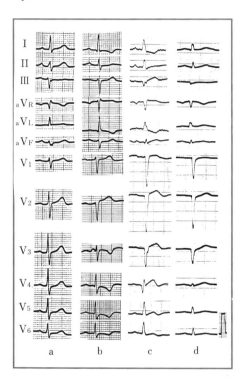

FIG. 201 Electrocardiograms. a: 2 years 10 months before death, on first admission; b: 1 year 8 months before death, on second admission; c: 31 days before death, on day of infarction, d: 26 days before death.

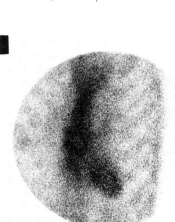

FIG. 202 ⁹⁹ᵐTc pyrophosphate myocardial scintigram. Frontal surface RI accumulation of ⁹⁹ᵐTc pyrophosphate throughout the surrounding myocardium is seen.

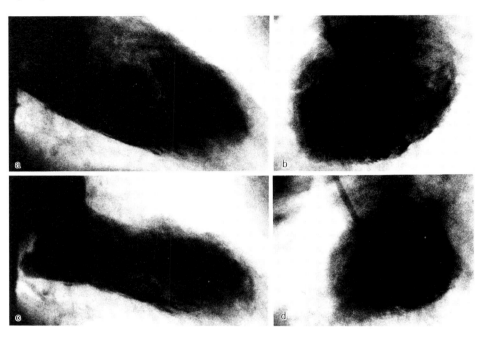

FIG. 203 Left ventriculography. a,b: diastole; c,d: systole.

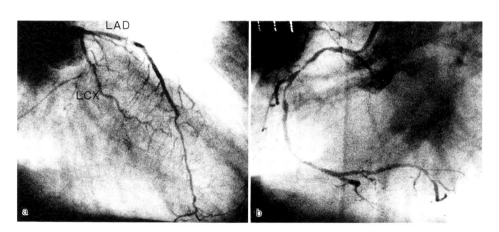

FIG. 204 Coronary angiography. One year 8 months before infarction. a: left coronary artery (LAD, left anterior descending artery; LCX, left circumflex artery); b: right coronary artery.

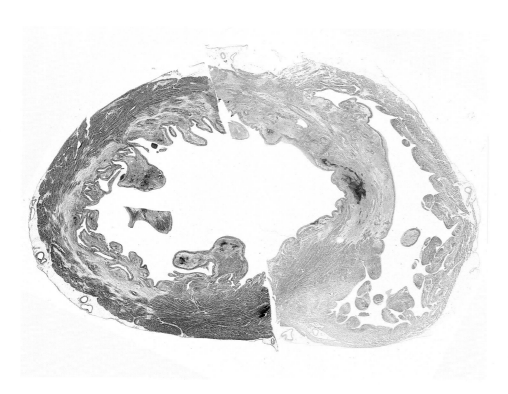

FIG. 225 Transverse histologic section. A transmural infarction with dense collagen fiber proliferation can be seen in the interventricular septum and anterior wall of the left ventricle. Light blue subendocardial fibrous areas are seen from the anterolateral wall to the posterior wall of the left ventricle. (Masson trichrome stain.)

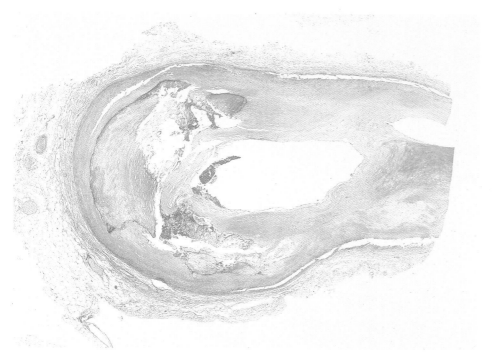

FIG. 228 Histologic findings in the left anterior descending artery (just after bifurcation of the left circumflex artery). The region marked with an arrow is shown in Fig. 227. An atheroma with calcification is evident, together with new mural thrombosis. (HE stain, × 17.)

Complications

FREE WALL RUPTURE

The second most common cause of death, following pump failure (cardiogenic shock) in acute myocardial infarction, is free wall rupture. At the National Cardiovascular Center, free wall rupture was found in 15 of 108 autopsies (14%) in which death was caused by acute myocardial infarction. The mean age of these 15 cases was 69 (51–83) years, which was 3 years older than in the nonrupture group. The percentage of females was also higher than in the nonrupture group.

Twelve of these 15 cases had a history of hypertension, suggesting that blood pressure control following acute myocardial infarction is an important factor in the prevention of rupture.

Almost all free wall ruptures occurred within 1 week after acute myocardial infarction, but two peaks were noted. The first occurred within 24 hours after infarction and the second after 3 to 7 days, suggesting that rupture is related to the serial tissue changes occurring in acute myocardial infarction. The high risk of cardiac ruptures during this period is attributed to myocardial tissue weakness, the infiltration of inflammatory cells such as neutrophils and macrophages, and the promotion of necrosis by various enzymes and chemical substances. Accordingly, cardiac rupture is unlikely to occur once fibrosis has progressed sufficiently.

Since free wall rupture is, of course, a complication of transmural infarction, the associated incidence of coronary thrombosis is also high. Lesions in one branch of the left anterior descending artery are present in the majority of cases, and the site of the rupture is typically the apex at the anterior wall of the left ventricle.

The types of rupture have been classified by Becker et al. as follows: type I: slit-like tears, type II: erosive progressive tears, and type III: aneurysmal formation. The majority of ruptures show distinct openings in the tissue.

VENTRICULAR SEPTAL RUPTURE

The incidence of ventricular septal rupture (perforation) associated with acute myocardial infarction is 1% to 2%. This complication has a poor prognosis and is associated with cardiogenic shock or severe bilateral heart failure. The mortality rate is 24% within 1 day and 65% within 2 weeks. The 2-month survival rate is 13%.

The only method of saving the patient's life is surgical closure of the rupture, but the results of surgery have been far from promising, with 39 of 80 patients dying in one multicenter study. However, more aggressive surgical approaches have recently resulted in improvement in survival.

Tables 6 and 7 summarize the clinical characteristics and autopsy findings in 7 patients with interventricular septal rupture studied at the National Cardiovascular Center. The mean age was 70.9 years, similar to that for free wall ruptures. Likewise, the number of women was higher than men, and all patients had a history of hypertension.

Table 6. Clinical characteristics in ventricular septal ruptures (VSR)

Case	Age	Sex	History Hypertension	Diabetes	Symptoms at onset	Onset to admission	Onset to VSR	Survival after IVSR	VFWR	Heart murmur	Shunt rate (%)	ECG findings	Enzymes SGOT	CK	LDH	Post infarction BP (mmHg)	Cause of death
1 CB	71	F	+	–	Chest pain	About 12 hours	<1 day	12 days	–	+	56	II, III, aVF: ST↑ V2–6, I, aVL: ST↓ III A-V block	282	2826	ND	78/48	Vtach→VF
2 TM	67	M	+	–	Chest pain	1 hour	No diagnosis within 10 hours	Died 10 hours after onset	–	–	ND	I, II, aVL, V2–6: ST↑ II, III, aVF, V1–6: Q(+)	304	1848	702	180–190/	Cardiogenic shock
3 SF	75	F	+	–	Chest pain	5 hours	8.5 hours	7.5 hours	+ (RV)	+	35	V1–4: QS, ST↑ V3–5: ST re-elevation	242	1944	732	166/96	Cardiogenic shock
4 IK	75	F	+	+	Chest pain	3 hours	6 days	60 days (operation)	–	+	61.7	I, aVL, V1–6: ST↑ II, III, aVF: ST↓ LBBB→III A-V block	812	4776	ND	102/70	Acute arrhythmia
5 KM	56	M	+	–	Chest pain	Hospitalized day of onset, transferred to Center after 12 days	9 days	7 days (operation)	+ (LV)	+	66	II, III, aVF: Q(+), ST↑, Tinvert	404	430	1245	112/86 9 days after onset	Tamponade
6 MN	77	M	+	+	Chest pain	2 hours	9 days	4 hours	–	+	85	II, III, aVF: ST↑ I, aVR, V2,3: ST↓	364	2568	1356	110/70	Cardiogenic shock
7 IT	75	M	+	–	Malaise	Hospitalized day of onset, transferred to Center after 10 days	10 days	38 days	–	+	36	V1–6: QS, ST↑	118 (changed hospital)	614	2192	100/70	Vtach→VF

Abbreviations: VFWR, ventricular free wall rupture; Vtach, ventricular tachycardia; VF, ventricular fibrillation; ND, not detected.

CASE 11 FREE WALL RUPTURE, ANTERIOR WALL INFARCTION (13 HOURS)

The patient was a 68-year-old man who smoked 20 to 30 cigarettes a day. He was hypertensive but not diabetic. Two years and 3 months before death, he noted chest discomfort on exertion. While recording the ECG, chest pain appeared, and ST segment depression was seen in leads I, $_aV_L$, and V_{4-6}. Unstable angina pectoris was diagnosed, and the patient was hospitalized. Left ventriculography and coronary angiography revealed 75% stenosis of segments 7 and 9 of the left anterior descending artery, and reduced contraction of the anterolateral wall. Mitral insufficiency was moderately severe, the left ventricular ejection fraction was 61%, and no further chest pain occurred after hospital discharge.

After taking a bath 13 hours before death, he felt precordial tightness, his face became pale, and orthopnea developed. He was admitted to the CCU 8 hours before death. On admission, his blood pressure was 136/110 mmHg, his pulse rate was 76 beats/min and irregular, WBC was 10,500/mm³, serum CK was 69 IU/L, and SGOT was 29 IU/L. On the ECG, ST segment elevation was noted in leads I, $_aV_L$, and V_{2-3}, ST segment depression in leads II, III, $_aV_F$, and V_{4-6}, and T wave inversion in leads V_{2-6}. The pulmonary artery wedge pressure was 14 mmHg and the cardiac index 1.56 L/min/m². The QRS axis suddenly changed on the monitor ECG 30 minutes before death, and a junctional rhythm appeared. Blood pressure measurement became impossible and cardiac rupture was diagnosed by echocardiography.

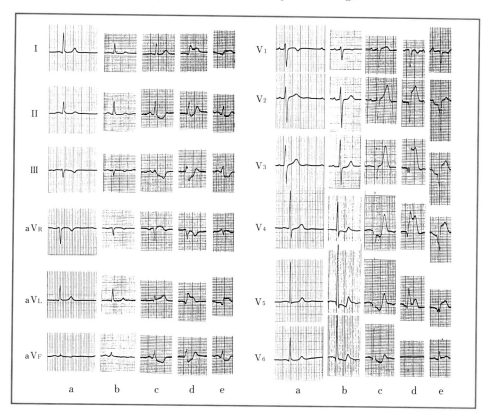

FIG. 234 Electrocardiograms. a: 1 year 1 month before death, before onset of infarction; b: 1 day before death, 1 hour after infarction; c: 2 hours after infarction; d: 5 hours before rupture; e: 20 minutes before death.

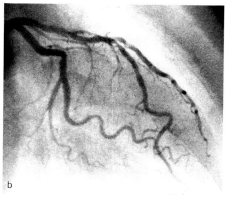

FIG. 235 Coronary angiography. a: right coronary artery before infarction; b: left coronary artery.

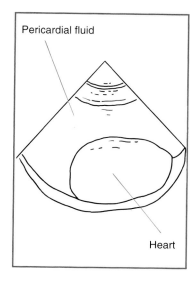

FIG. 236 Echocardiogram. Extensive accumulation of pericardial fluid surrounded the heart.

Pericardial fluid

Heart

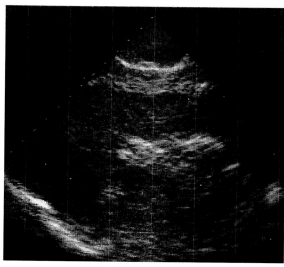

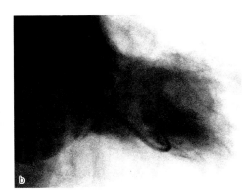

FIG. 237 Left ventriculography. a: end-diastole; b: end-systole.

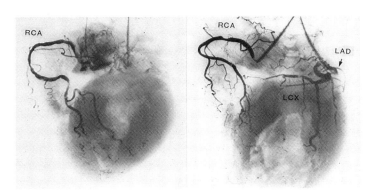

FIG. 238 Postmortem angiography. (LAD, left anterior descending artery; LCX, left circumflex artery; RCA, right coronary artery.)

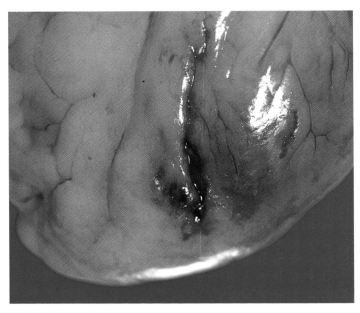

FIG. 240 Ruptured area. A rupture of about 2.5 cm is present in the apex, and bleeding is seen in the surrounding tissue.

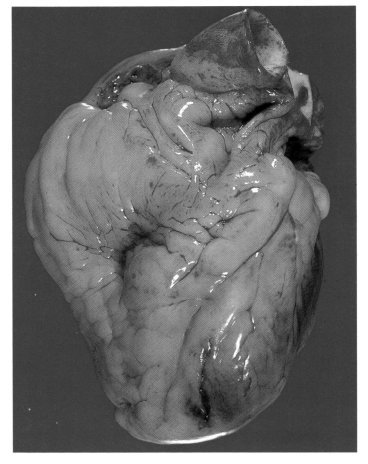

FIG. 239 Frontal surface of the heart. Heart weight: 410 g. The apex consists of the left ventricle (60%) and the right ventricle (40%). The anterior wall of the left ventricle has changed to a reddish-brown color, with petechial hemorrhages present subepicardially. A rupture of about 2.5 cm is present in the apex.

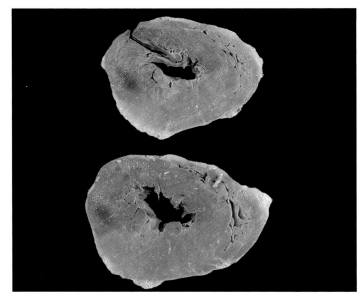

FIG. 241 Transverse sections. Level of one-third from the apex. Discoloration is evident in the anterior portion of the interventricular septum and the anterolateral wall of the left ventricle. A comparatively sharp rupture is present in the anterior wall of the left ventricle and the area of transition into the interventricular septum. Small hemorrhagic foci are present in the surrounding tissue.

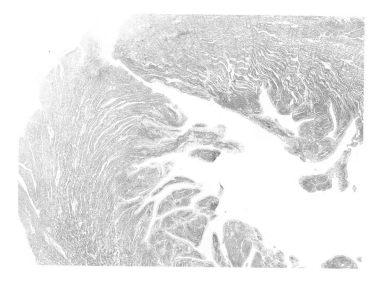

FIG. 242 Transverse histologic section. A rupture exists in the anterior wall of the left ventricle and the area of transition into the interventricular septum. Myocardial fibers in the anterior wall and anterior portion of the interventricular septum show wavy changes and hemorrhage. (HE stain, × 3.)

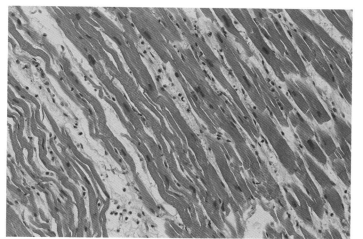

FIG. 243 Histologic findings in the infarcted area. The myocardial fibers show eosinophilic staining and are attenuated and wavy. Karyopyknosis and contraction band necrosis are also present. The interstitium is edematous and neutrophil infiltration is evident. (HE stain, × 180.)

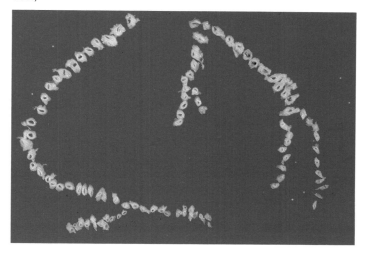

FIG. 244 Coronary arteries. Complete occlusion resulting from hemorrhage in the atheroma and thrombi are seen in the proximal part (segment 6) of the left anterior descending artery. Significant stenosis is not present in the right coronary artery or left circumflex artery.

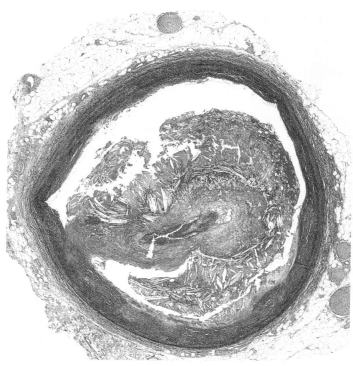

FIG. 245 Histologic findings in the proximal part of the left anterior descending artery (segment 6). Complete occlusion resulting from an atheroma and mural thrombus is evident. (Masson trichrome elastica van Gieson stain, × 16.)

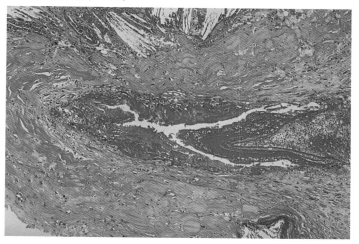

FIG. 246 Histologic finding of the left anterior descending artery (segment 6). Complete occlusion caused by mural thrombi is seen. (HE stain, × 65.)

Left Ventricular Infarction   105

CASE 12 VENTRICULAR SEPTAL RUPTURE

The patient was an 81-year-old woman with hypertension and diabetes. Nine days before death, chest pains appeared at rest. Fifteen hours before death, the patient had chest pain associated with cold sweat. She was examined by a local physician 13 hours before death. Q wave development was noted in leads V_{1-3} and ST segment elevation in leads V_{1-4} on ECG. She was hospitalized 9 hours before death. On admission, her blood pressure was 120/70 mmHg and pulse rate was 70 beats/min and regular. The WBC was 9,200/mm^3, serum CK 846 IU/L, and SGOT 118 IU/L. Echocardiography and flow color Doppler imaging revealed no contraction of the anterior wall, and the presence of an interventricular septal rupture. An intra-aortic balloon pumping (IABP) device was inserted because of cardiogenic shock, but ventricular fibrillation occurred repeatedly, and the patient died.

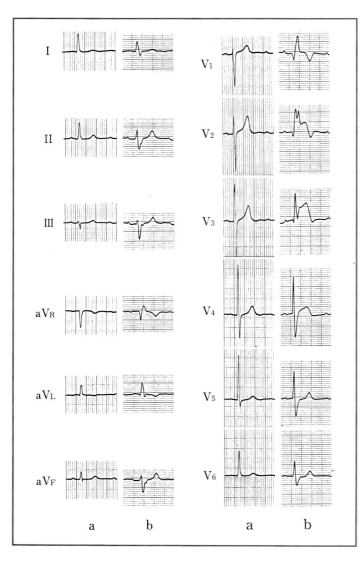

FIG. 247 Electrocardiograms. a: before the infarction; 4 years before death; b: 13 hours before death.

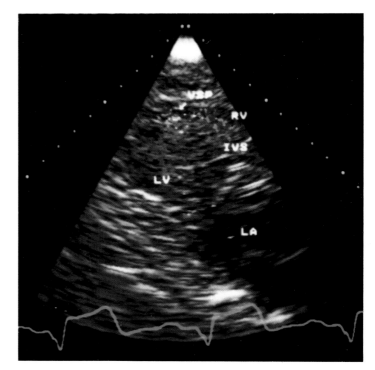

FIG. 248 Color Doppler method. Blood flow from the left to right ventricle (arrow) shows a mosaic pattern. (IVS, interventricular septum; LA, left atrium; LV, left ventricle; RV, right ventricle; VSP, interventricular septal rupture.)

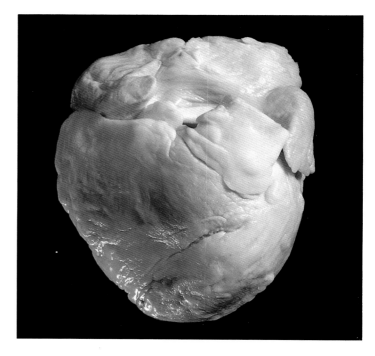

FIG. 249 Frontal surface of the heart. Heart weight: 420 g. Marked enlargement of the four chambers is evident, and the heart is spherical.

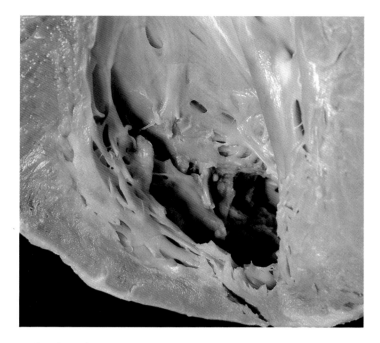

FIG. 250 Left ventricular surface of the interventricular septum. A rupture of about 1 cm in diameter is seen in the apex. Thrombi adhere to the ruptured area. Extensive discoloration and rupture of the trabeculae carneae cordis are seen in the anterior wall of the left ventricle.

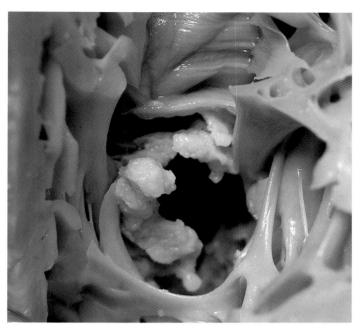

FIG. 251 Right ventricular surface of the interventricular septum. A rupture is seen in the apex. Thrombi adhere to the margin of the rupture.

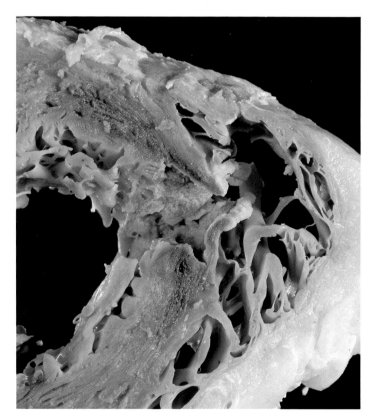

FIG. 252 Transverse section of the interventricular septum. A rupture is seen at a site about one-third from the posterior wall of the interventricular septum. White thrombi adhere to the ruptured region and hemorrhage is also evident.

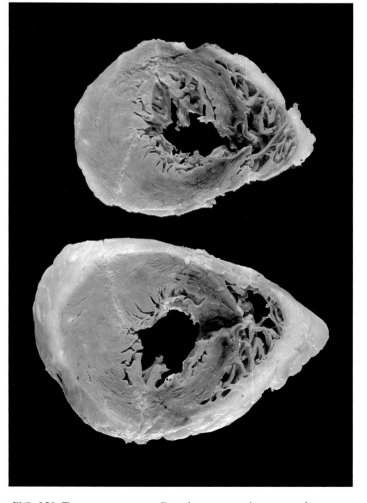

FIG. 253 Transverse sections. Discoloration can be seen in the anterior wall of the left ventricle, the interventricular septum, and part of the posterior wall. Perforation associated with hemorrhage is noted about one-third of the distance from the posterior wall of the septum. The septum is rather thin.

Left Ventricular Infarction   107

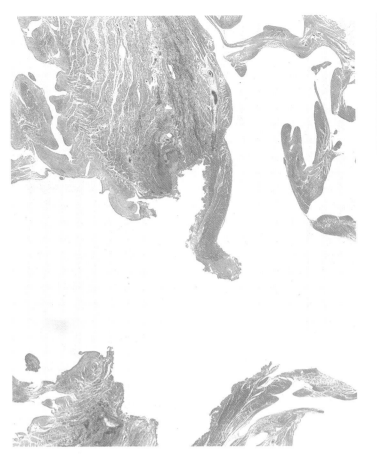

FIG. 254 Histologic findings in the interventricular septal rupture. Myocardial fibers show wavy changes. Hemorrhage and the adhesion of thrombi are present in the ruptured area. (HE stain, × 5.7.)

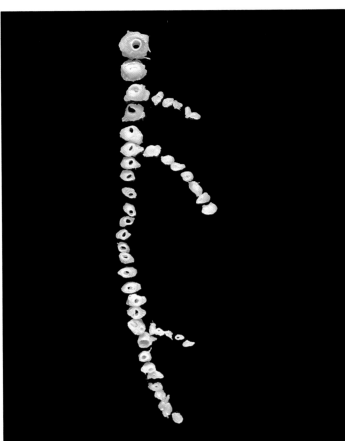

FIG. 255 Right coronary artery. Severe stenosis of more than 90% is noted in the proximal area. Hypoplasia of the right coronary artery is evident.

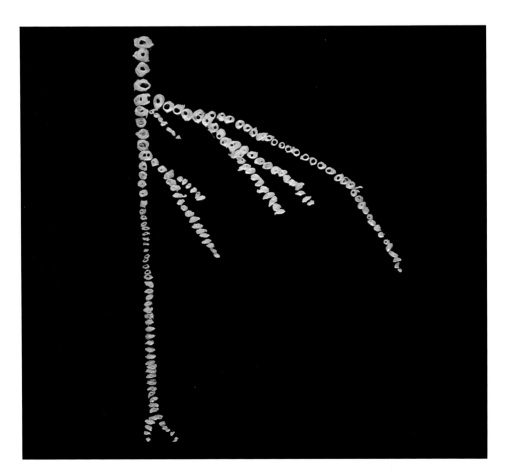

FIG. 256 Left coronary artery. Stenosis resulting from an atheroma and thrombotic occlusion is seen in the proximal portion of the left anterior descending artery. Severe stenosis of more than 90% is found in the distal portion of the left circumflex artery.

CASE 14 INTERVENTRICULAR SEPTAL RUPTURE, FREE WALL RUPTURE (2 DAYS)

The patient was a 75-year-old woman who smoked 10 cigarettes a day. She was hypertensive but not diabetic. About 48 hours before death, she developed precordial distress, dyspnea, and vomiting. Dyspnea continued for more than 10 hours. About 22 hours before death, the feeling of precordial distress recurred and gradually intensified, peaking 16 hours before death. The patient was admitted to the CCU 9 hours before death. On admission, her blood pressure was 166/96 mmHg, and her pulse rate was 76 beats/min and regular. Rales were heard in both lower lung fields. The serum CK was 1,088 IU/L and the SGOT 114 IU/L. In the ECG, QS patterns and ST segment elevation were noted in leads V$_{1-4}$. The mean pulmonary artery wedge pressure was 15 mmHg, mean left atrial pressure 5 mmHg, and cardiac index 2.43 L/min/m^2 (Forrester I). About 8 hours before death, her blood pressure fell to 100/80 mmHg, and a pansystolic murmur (4/6), most intense between the third and fourth ribs at the left margin of the left sternum, was heard. An interventricular septal rupture was diagnosed. The patient suddenly began to moan 50 minutes before death and became unconscious. Respiratory arrest occurred, leading to death.

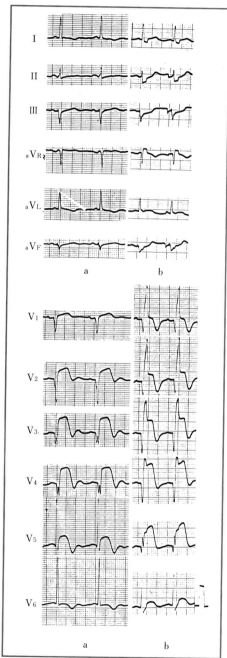

FIG. 271 Electrocardiograms. a: 9 hours before death; b: 5 hours before death.

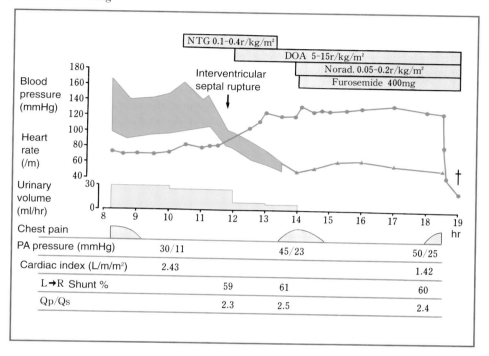

FIG. 272 Clinical course. (PA, pulmonary artery.)

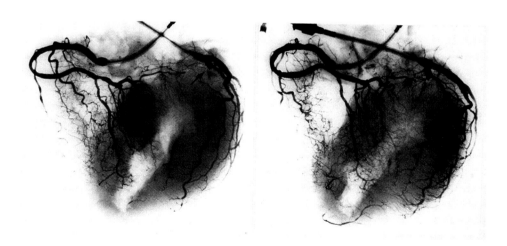

FIG. 273 Postmortem angiography.

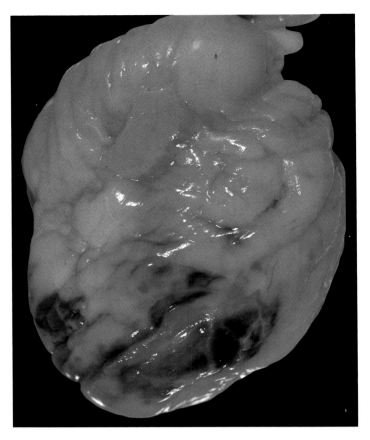

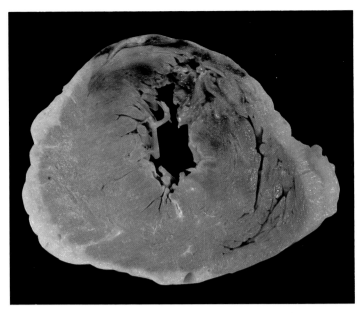

FIG. 275 Transverse section. Discoloration is evident in the anterior portion of the interventricular septum and the anterior wall of the left ventricle. A rupture can be seen near the transition region from the interventricular septum to the left ventricle. Part of the right ventricular wall is eroded and hemorrhage can be seen in the epicardium.

FIG. 274 Front surface of the heart. Heart weight: 410 g. Hemorrhage and fissures are seen in the apex.

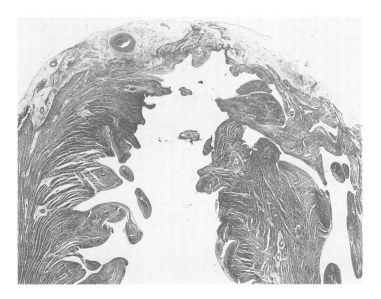

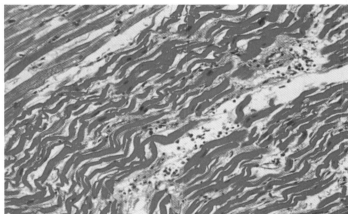

FIG. 277 Histologic findings in the infarcted area. The myocardial fibers are dissociated and eosinophilic. Striations have disappeared, karyopyknosis is present, and some denucleation is found. The interstitium is edematous and marked neutrophil infiltration is evident. (HE stain, × 130.)

FIG. 276 Transverse histologic section. A rupture is evident near the region of transition from the interventricular septum to the left ventricle. A tear in the myocardium of the right ventricular wall and hemorrhage into the epicardium are present. (HE stain, × 3.5.)

FIG. 291 Transverse histologic section. Dense collagen fiber hyperplasia is seen throughout the entire circumference of the left ventricle. Red mural thrombi can be noted in the anterior wall. (Masson trichrome stain.)

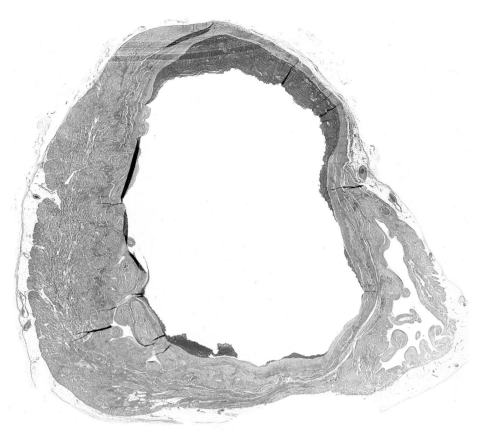

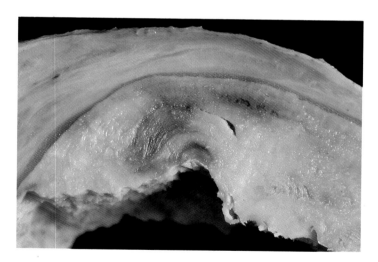

FIG. 292 Intraventricular thrombosis. The anterior wall of the left ventricle is white, gelatinous, and thin. A lamellar structure is evident in the thrombus.

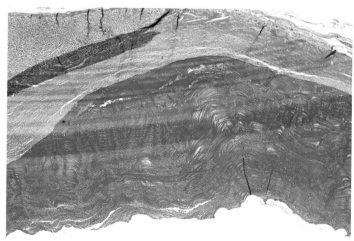

FIG. 293 Histologic findings in the thrombus. The anterior wall of the left ventricle consists entirely of blue collagen fibers. A lamellar structure is noted in the reddish-violet mural thrombus. (Masson trichrome stain, × 8.5.)

Case 16 Cardiac Aneurysm, Inferior Wall Infarction (5 months)

The patient was a 66-year-old man who smoked five cigarettes a day. He was hypertensive and diabetic. He had gout and hypertension for 13 years before death. A cerebral infarction occurred 3 years before death. About 1 year before death, the patient felt chest discomfort on exertion. Five months before death, the patient developed a cold sweat and nausea while watching television, and he was admitted to a local hospital with a diagnosis of myocardial infarction. Because of frequent episodes of ventricular tachycardia, he changed hospitals 3 months before death. His mean pulmonary artery wedge pressure was 4 mmHg and cardiac index 2.1 L/min/m². The ventricular tachycardia was controlled by drugs such as procainamide, but he was switched to phenytoin because of a skin rash. Three hours before death, cold sweat, nausea, and vomiting appeared, and the patient's blood pressure fell. The patient did not respond to treatment and died.

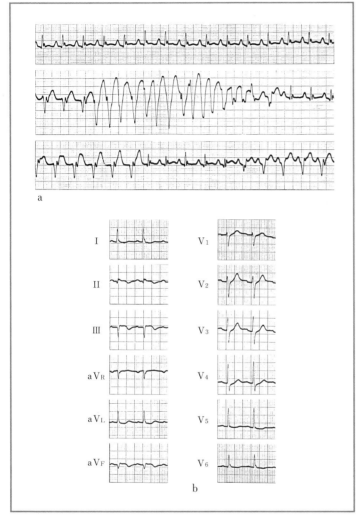

FIG. 294 Electrocardiograms. a: monitor ECG, onset on ventricular tachycardia; b: control.

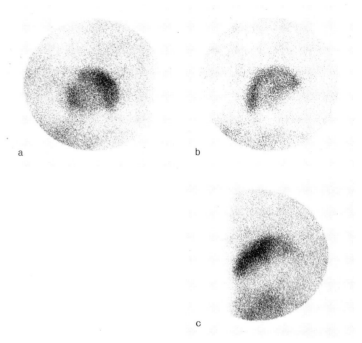

FIG. 295 Myocardial scintigrams. a: frontal aspect; b: left anterior oblique 45° aspect; c: lateral aspect. Extensive defect images are seen from the inferior to the posterior wall.

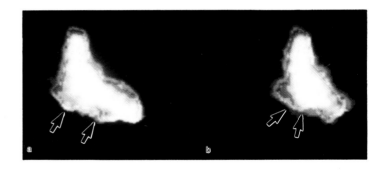

FIG. 296 Gated blood-pool scintigram using ⁹⁹ᵐTc-labeled erythrocytes. Right anterior oblique 30° aspect. a: end-diastole; b: end-systole. A cardiac aneurysm (arrow) is seen in the inferoposterior wall.

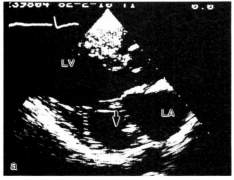
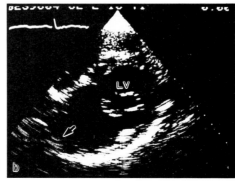

FIG 297 Two-dimensional echocardiograms. a: long-axis two-dimensional echocardiogram; b: short-axis two-dimensional echocardiogram. Formation of a cardiac aneurysm (arrow) is seen in the posterior wall. (LA, left atrium; LV, left ventricle.)

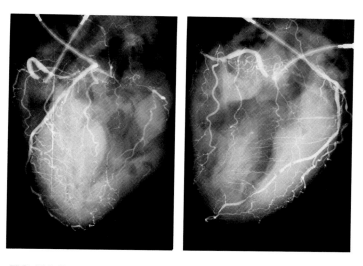

FIG. 298 Postmortem angiography.

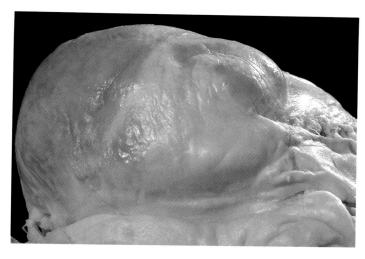

FIG. 299 Cardiac aneurysm in the posterior wall of the left ventricle. Heart weight: 470 g. The wall has become thin and an aneurysmal protrusion is seen on its surface.

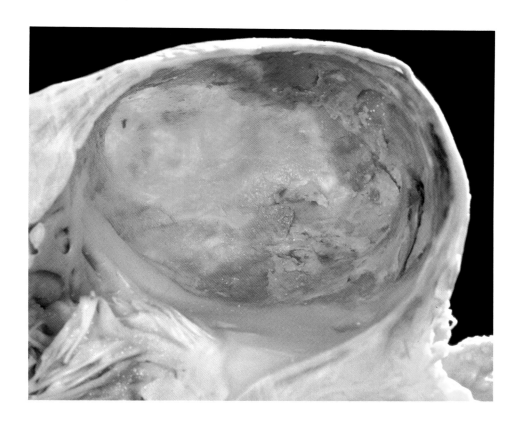

FIG. 300 Cardiac aneurysm. The posterior wall of the left ventricle is thin and consists only of fibrous connective tissue. An aneurysm has formed, and mural thrombi adhere to its inner surface.

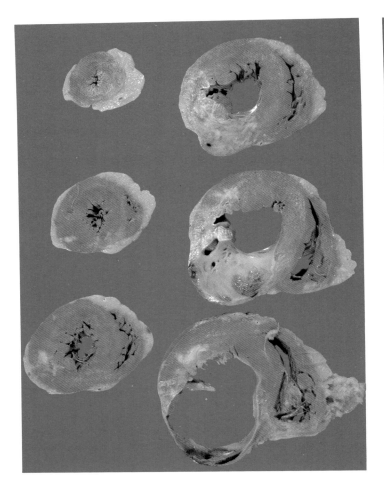

FIG. 301 Transverse sections. Thinning of the posterior wall of the left ventricle and formation of an aneurysm are seen from the level of the tendinous cords to that of the center of the papillary muscles. Fibrosis is present in the anterior wall.

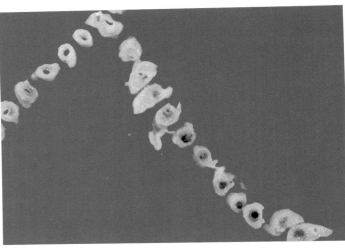

FIG. 303 Left coronary artery. Marked stenosis is seen from just after bifurcation.

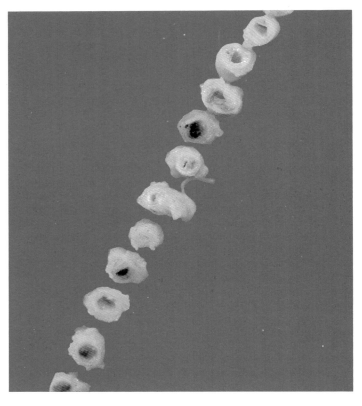

FIG. 302 Right coronary artery. Severe stenosis resulting from an atheroma is seen in segment 2.

CASE 17 CARDIAC ANEURYSMECTOMY

The patient was a 63-year-old man who smoked 20 cigarettes a day. He was hypertensive but not diabetic. The patient was hospitalized in a local hospital for an anteroseptal myocardial infarction 3 years 11 months before death. Because of progressive heart failure, he was transferred to the National Cardiovascular Center 3 years 10 months before death. Left ventriculography and coronary angiography revealed 90% stenosis of segment 6 of the left anterior descending artery, abnormal contraction of the anterolateral wall and apex, and weakened contraction of the anterior basal and diaphragmatic walls. The ejection fraction was 21%. Left cardiac aneurysmectomy was performed 3 years 6 months before death. After discharge, heart failure developed, and the patient had repeated episodes of deterioration and improvement, but he died of an acute subdural hematoma.

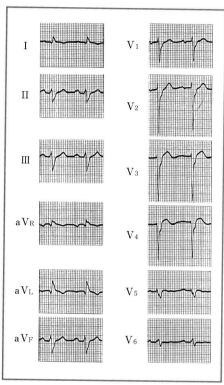

FIG. 304 Electrocardiogram recorded on admission.

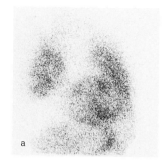 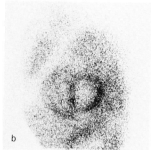 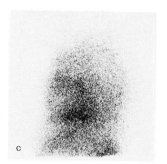

FIG. 305 Myocardial scintigrams. a: frontal aspect; b: left anterior oblique 45° aspect; c: left lateral aspect. Extensive defects can be seen from the apex to the anterior wall, the left ventricle is clearly imaged, and thallium is increased in the lung field. Heart failure is suspected.

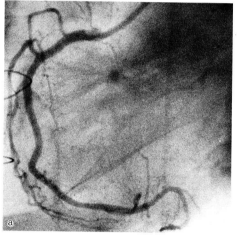 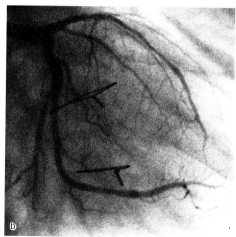

FIG. 306 Postoperative coronary angiography. a: right coronary artery, b: left coronary artery.

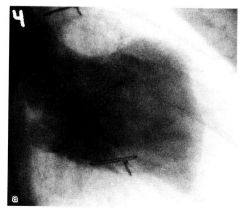 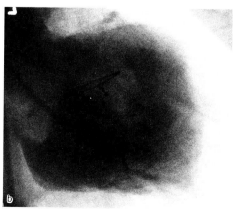

FIG. 307 Postoperative left ventriculography. a: end-systole; b: end-diastole.

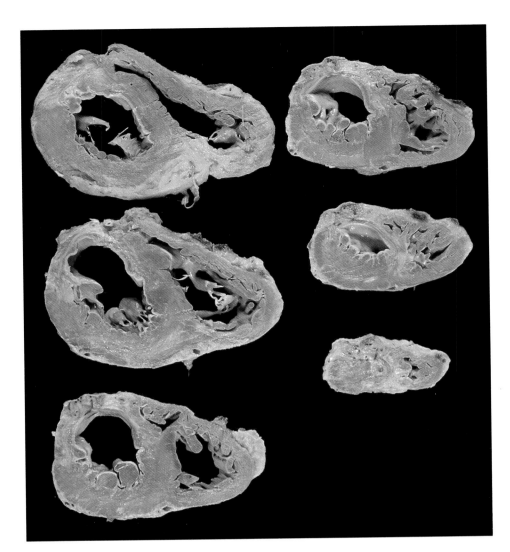

FIG. 308 Transverse sections. A white old myocardial infarction is seen in the anterior wall of the left ventricle and anterior part of the interventricular septum from the level of the tendinous cords to the apex. The walls are thin and the ventricular cavity is enlarged. Fibrosis is seen in the posterolateral wall. Blue surgical thread is present from the level of the center of the papillary muscles to the apex of the heart.

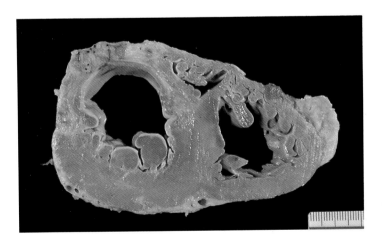

FIG. 309 Transverse section. Level of the center of the papillary muscles. Translucent white fibrosis can be seen in the anterior portion of the interventricular septum and the anterior wall of the left ventricle. Blue surgical thread is present in the anterior wall. Sporadic fibrosis is also observed in the posterior wall.

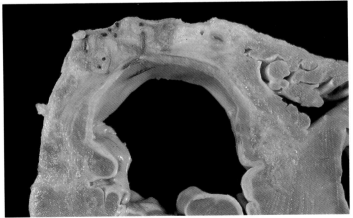

FIG. 310 Close-up view of the infarcted area. A translucent white old infarction is evident, together with marked fibrous thickening of the endocardium. Blue surgical thread is present.

CASE 18 PAPILLARY MUSCLE DYSFUNCTION, ANTERIOR WALL INFARCTION (1 YEAR 3 MONTHS)

The patient was a 60-year-old woman who was not hypertensive or diabetic. One year 3 months before death, she developed nocturnal dyspnea and chest discomfort. A local physician diagnosed heart failure and liver dysfunction. Ten months before death, an old myocardial infarction and hyperlipemia were diagnosed, and she was treated as an outpatient. The patient was hospitalized for heart failure 7 months before death. On flow Doppler imaging, moderately severe mitral insufficiency and mild to moderate tricuspid insufficiency were found. On RI angiography, the left ventricular ejection fraction was 18%, and the right ventricular ejection rate was 35%. Coronary angiography revealed complete occlusion of segment 7 of the left anterior descending artery. Two months before death, the patient was hospitalized for a recurrence of heart failure. Despite treatment, the heart failure gradually worsened, and the patient died.

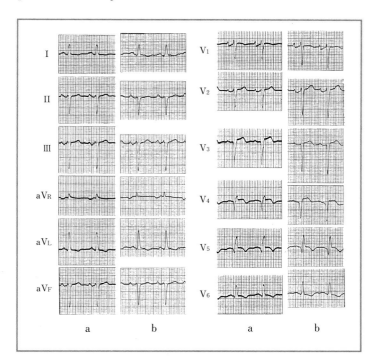

FIG. 311 Electrocardiograms. a: 7 months before; b: 48 days before.

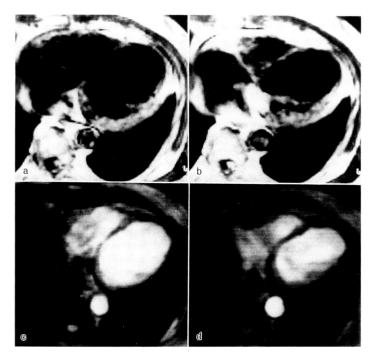

FIG. 312 ECG-synchronized MRI. a,c: end-diastole; b,d: end-systole; a,b: ECG-synchronized spin-echo method; c,d: cine magnetic resonance method. Thinning of the wall is seen from the anterior wall to the apex. Overall contractility of the heart has declined, coincident with heart failure.

FIG. 313 Two-dimensional echocardiogram. a: long-axis two-dimensional echocardiogram; b: short-axis two-dimensional echocardiogram at the level of the papillary muscles. Thinning of the interventricular septum and anterior wall and enlargement of the left ventricular chamber are evident. (LA, left atrium; LV, left ventricle.)

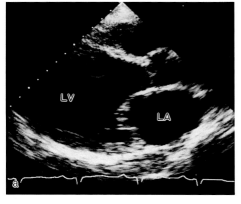

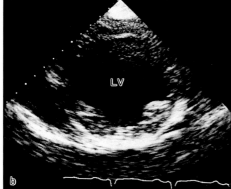

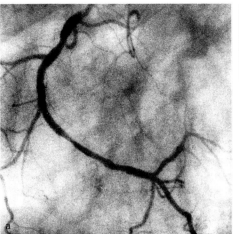 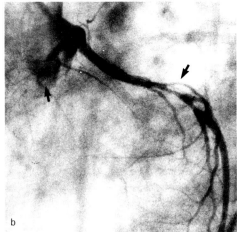 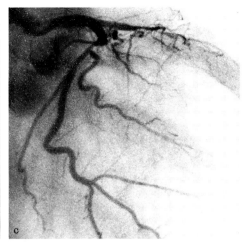

FIG. 314 Coronary angiography. a: right coronary artery; b: left anterior oblique aspect of the left coronary artery; c: right anterior oblique aspect of the left coronary artery.

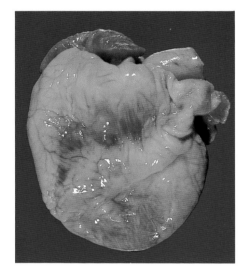

FIG. 315 Frontal surface of the heart. Heart weight: 500 g. Thinning of the anterolateral wall of the left ventricle is noted and the heart is spherical.

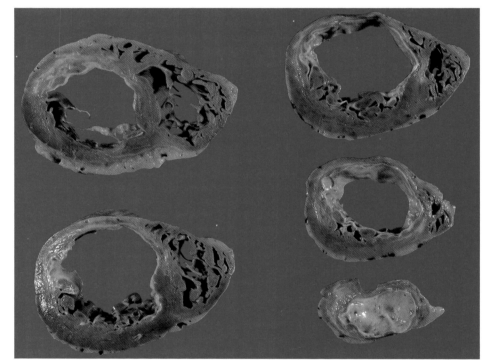

FIG. 316 Transverse sections. Thinning of the anterior portion of the interventricular septum and anterolateral wall of the left ventricle can be seen from the level of the tendinous cords through the apex. The ventricular cavity shows aneurysmal enlargement.

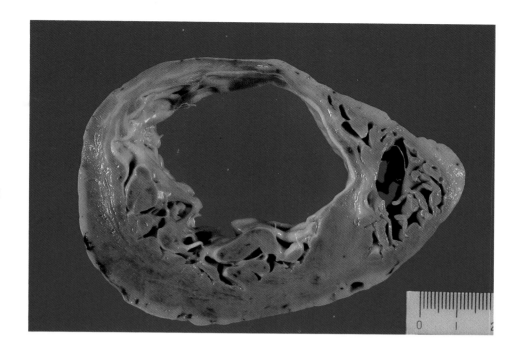

FIG. 317 Transverse section. Level of the center of the papillary muscles. Fibrosis and thinning are present from the anterior portion of the interventricular septum to the anterolateral wall of the left ventricle. Fibrous hypertrophy of the endocardium is noted. Part of the anterolateral papillary muscles show fibrosis and thinning.

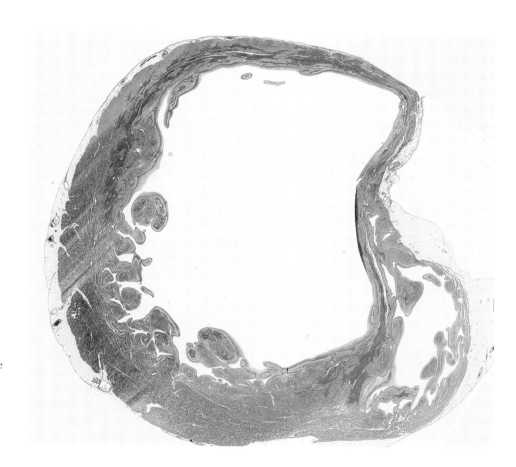

FIG. 318 Histologic transverse section. The interventricular septum and anterolateral wall of the left ventricle are almost completely replaced by fibrous tissue and show thinning. (Masson trichrome stain.)

Arrhythmia

Arrhythmia is the most frequent complication of acute myocardial infarction, and there are many types of arrhythmia (Figs. 319 and 320). However, the development and widespread availability of CCUs in recent years have contributed to a sharp decline in mortality because of arrhythmias, which previously ranked behind pump failure. Nonetheless, arrhythmia remains the prime cause of death in many patients with acute myocardial infarction who die within 1 hour after the onset of symptoms before hospitalization.

Research on arrhythmias occurring in experimental models of myocardial infarction indicates that ventricular extrasystoles and ventricular tachycardia develop within 15 to 30 minutes (Harris Phase 1) after coronary artery occlusion, frequently leading to ventricular flutter. In the period between 4 to 8 hours and 24 to 48 hours after occlusion (Harris Phase 2), ventricular tachycardia or idioventricular rhythm appears. Ventricular extrasystoles and ventricular tachycardia are most likely to occur 3 to 10 days after coronary artery occlusion. The mechanism involved in the onset of arrhythmia in myocardial infarction is theorized to be (1) reentry, (2) increased ectopic automaticity, or (3) both of these factors. Surgical treatment such as (1) resection of the infarcted area, (2) resection of the endocardium, (3) endomyocardial coronary incision, and (4) cryoablation is indicated in intractable ventricular tachycardia associated with reentry.

Coronary artery reconstruction such as coronary artery bypass grafting may be effective against arrhythmias that are produced by ischemic episodes.

Pump Failure

In acute myocardial infarction, various degrees of pump failure, directly proportional to the extent of myocardial necrosis, occur because of compromised left ventricular function and reduced left ventricular diastolic compliance. Pump failure is the leading cause of death in acute myocardial infarction. In particular, the mortality rate exceeds 80% in cases complicated by cardiogenic

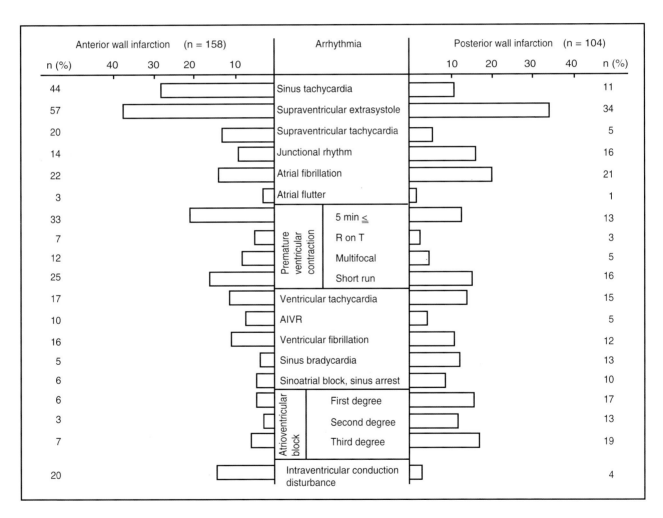

FIG. 319 Incidence of various arrhythmias in anterior and posterior wall infarctions. (From Kasanuki H: Myocardial infarctions: complications. Byori to Rinsho :4, 1986, with permission.)

shock occurring in the wake of severe pump failure. The clinical severity of pump failure may be expressed by the Killip (Table 4) and Forrester (Fig. 62) classifications.

PERICARDITIS

Clinically, pericarditis has been reported to occur as a complication in 7% to 16% of cases of acute myocardial infarction, but it is found with a higher prevalence at autopsy. Pericarditis typically appears 2 to 3 days after onset of transmural myocardial infarction and then disappears from several hours to 1 to 2 days later. Localized pericarditis develops into generalized pericarditis in about 10% of cases, and this leads to accumulation of pericardial fluid. However, development of constrictive pericarditis is rare.

The *Dressler syndrome* is a general term applied to pericarditis and pleurisy, which occurs 2 to 10 weeks after myocardial infarction. It is associated with nonspecific inflammatory findings, such as fever and leukocytosis, and pleuritic chest pain.

MURAL THROMBOSIS

At autopsy, mural thrombosis is associated with myocardial infarction in 44% of cases. Clinically, the detection rate by two-dimensional echocardiography or left ventriculography is reportedly 17% to 41%. Transesophageal echocardiography is more sensitive in its ability to detect mural left ventricular and left atrial thrombi.

Mural thrombosis is a frequent complication of anterior wall infarction, but is rarely associated with inferoposterior wall infarction. The most common site of mural thrombosis is the apex of the heart.

Arterial embolism caused by mural thrombosis occurs in 3% to 5% of all myocardial infarctions, and half of these cases suffer cerebral thromboembolism.

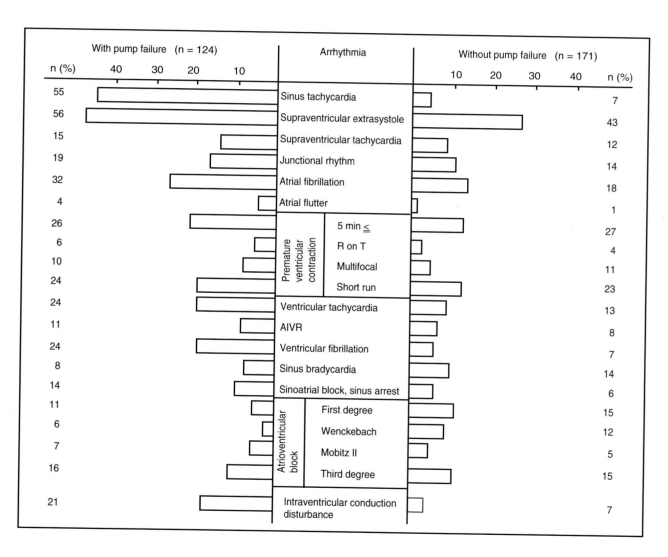

FIG. 320 Incidence of various arrhythmias in cases with and without pump failure. (From Kasanuki H: Myocardial infarctions: complications. Byori to Rinsho:4, 1986, with permission.)

Case 19 Heart Failure, Anterior Wall Infarction (11 years)

The patient was a 49-year-old man who smoked but was not hypertensive or diabetic. He suffered an anteroseptal wall infarction 11 years before death. Thereafter, mild dyspnea appeared on effort. About 18 months before death, exertional dyspnea intensified and angina pectoris developed. The patient was hospitalized 1 year 2 months before death for heart failure. The cardiothoracic ratio was 57%. On color flow Doppler imaging, mitral insufficiency was mild to moderate, and tricuspid insufficiency was severe. Left ventriculography and coronary angiography revealed 75% stenosis of the left main trunk and complete occlusion of segment 6 of the left anterior descending artery. No contraction was noted in the apex, the anterolateral, diaphragmatic, septal, or posterolateral walls, and weakened contraction was seen in the anterior and posterior basal walls. The ejection fraction was 11%. Surgery was not indicated and conservative treatment was continued. The NYHA cardiac function classification was 3 to 4. One month before death, the patient's heart failure worsened and he was readmitted. His condition was slightly improved by treatment, but ventricular fibrillation occurred and he died.

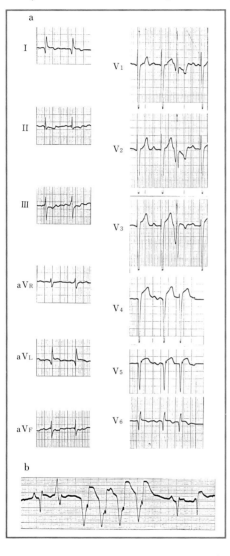

FIG. 321 Electrocardiograms. a: 1 year 2 months before death; b: 21 days before death.

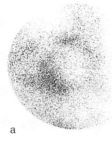
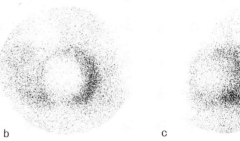

FIG. 322 Myocardial scintigrams. a: frontal aspect; b: left anterior oblique 45° aspect; c: lateral aspect. The heart chamber is enlarged, and void regions are seen from the anterior wall to the apex. Thallium activity is high in the lung fields, and heart failure is present as a complication.

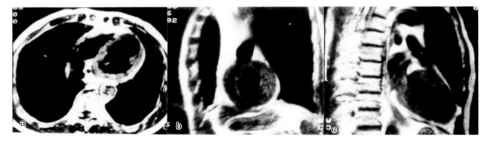

FIG. 323 ECG-synchronized MRI. a: body axis tomogram; b: short-axis tomogram; c: long-axis tomogram. Marked thinning of the wall is evident from the anterior wall to the apex.

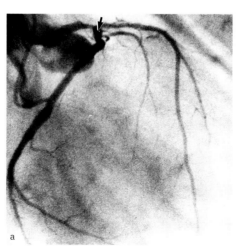
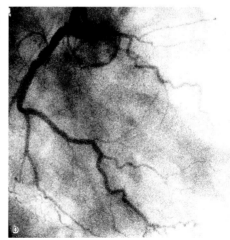

FIG. 324 Coronary angiography. a: right coronary artery; b: left coronary artery.

FIG. 325 Left ventriculography. a: end-systole; b: end-diastole.

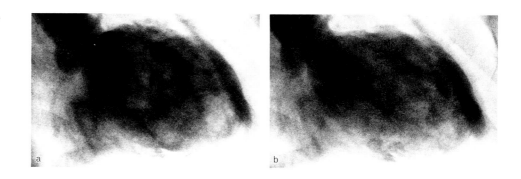

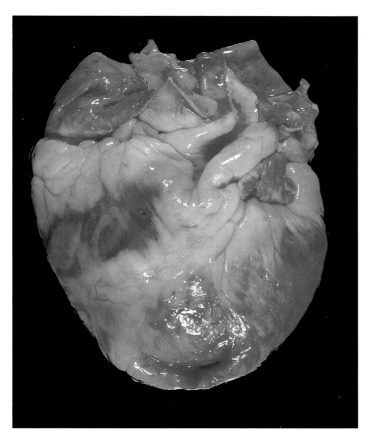

FIG. 326 Front surface of the heart. Heart weight: 615 g. The anterolateral wall of the left ventricle shows aneurysmal enlargement and the heart is spherical. Fibrous epicarditis is seen in the anterolateral wall of the left ventricle, thinning is especially prominent in the apex, and part of the wall is depressed into the chamber.

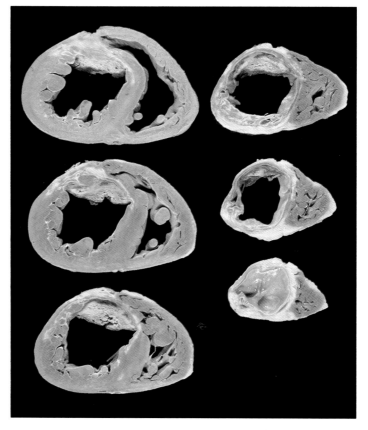

FIG. 327 Transverse sections. White fibrosis is evident in the anterior wall of the left ventricle and anterior portion of the interventricular septum from the level of the center of the papillary muscles to the apex. The fibrosis extends throughout the entire circumference of the left ventricle near the apex. The anterior wall and apex show thinning and marked enlargement. A mural thrombus is also evident.

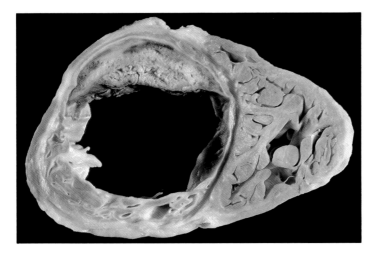

FIG. 328 Transverse section. Level about one-third from the apex. Fibrosis extends throughout the entire circumference of the left ventricle, and the ventricular chamber is enlarged. A mural thrombus adheres to the anterior wall.

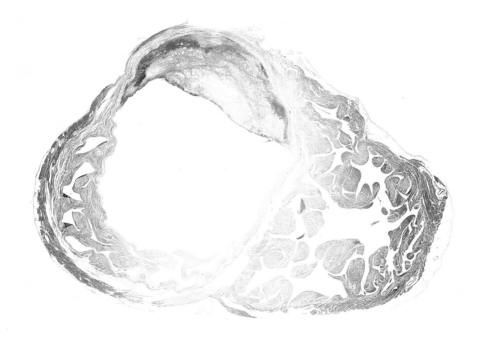

FIG. 329 Transverse histologic section. Fibrosis extends throughout the entire circumference of the left ventricle. Viable myocardium remains epicardially in the lateral and posterior walls. A mural thrombus adheres to the anterior wall.

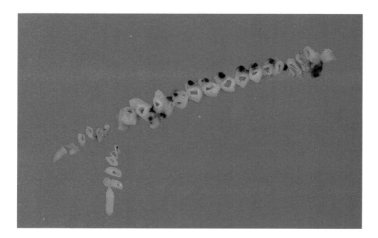

FIG. 330 Right coronary artery. The right coronary artery is hypoplastic.

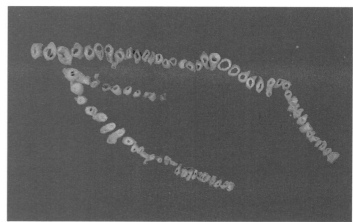

FIG. 331 Left coronary artery. Segment 6 of the left anterior descending artery is completely occluded. Significant stenosis is not seen in the left circumflex artery.

Case 20 Arrhythmia (Atrioventricular Block), Anterior Wall Infarction (13 days)

The patient was an 80-year-old woman who was hypertensive but not diabetic. She had been treated by a local physician for angina pectoris for 14 to 15 years. Atrial fibrillation was noted 4 years before death, and the patient was admitted because of a cerebral infarction 2 years 4 months before death. At about 5 AM, 13 days before death, the patient awoke because of chest pain, which recurred at about 5PM, 12 days before death. She was admitted to the CCU 11 days before death with a diagnosis of myocardial infarction. On admission, her blood pressure was 92/60 mmHg and pulse rate was 80 beats/min. Atrial fibrillation was present, and the WBC was 11,400/mm^3, serum CK 1,621 IU/L, and SGOT 422 IU/L. On the ECG, complete right bundle branch block, abnormal Q waves in leads III, $_aV_F$, and V_{1-3} and ST segment elevation and negative T waves in lead V_{3-6} were noted. CK activity reached a maximum value of 3,696 IU/L and SGOT 943 IU/L. Eleven days before death complete

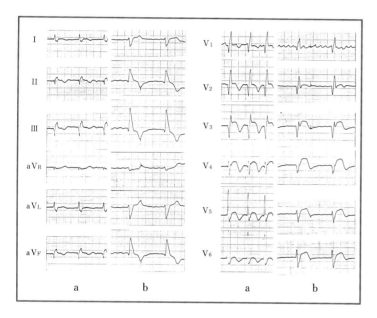

FIG. 332 Electrocardiograms. a: 11 days before, 2 days after onset of infarction, at admission; b: 10 days before, pacemaker rhythm.

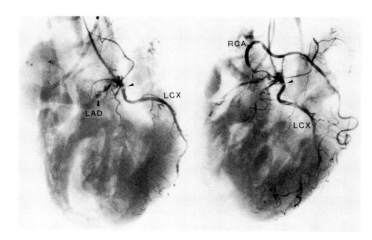

FIG. 333 Postmortem angiography. (LAD, left anterior descending artery; LCX, left circumflex artery; RCA, right coronary artery.)

atrioventricular block occurred at night and a pacemaker was implanted. The systolic murmur intensified and interventricular

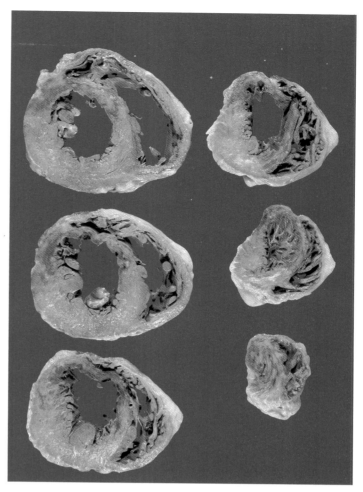

FIG. 334 Transverse sections. Heart weight: 500 g. Thinning and discoloration are seen in the anterior portion of the interventricular septum and anterior wall of the left ventricle from the base to the apex of the heart. An interventricular septal rupture is present about one-third from the apex.

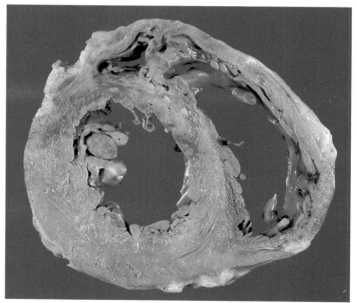

FIG. 335 Transverse section. Level of the tip of the papillary muscles. Discoloration is evident in the anterior portion of the interventricular septum and anterior wall of the left ventricle.

septal rupture was suspected 6 days before death. Thereafter, her blood pressure gradually fell and she died.

Left Ventricular Infarction 133

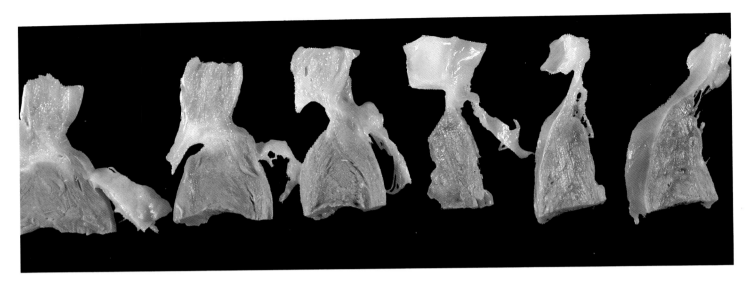

FIG. 336 Serial sections of the interventricular septum from the atrioventricular node to the junction of the left and right bundle branches. Discoloration can be seen at the junction of the left and right bundle branches and up to the atrioventricular ring in sections after the junction. No marked changes are seen in the atrioventricular node or near the bundle of His.

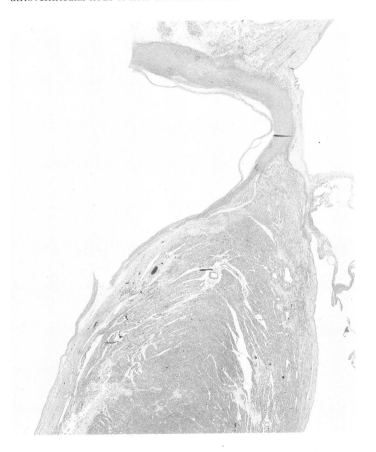

FIG. 337 Histologic findings in the conduction system. An infarcted area can be noted near the left bundle branch. (Masson trichrome stain, × 6.)

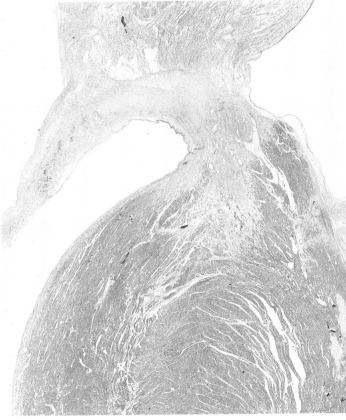

FIG. 338 Histologic findings in the conduction system (site of the penetrating bundle). An infarcted area is seen in the interventricular septum, but it does not reach the penetrating bundle. (Masson trichrome stain, × 6.)

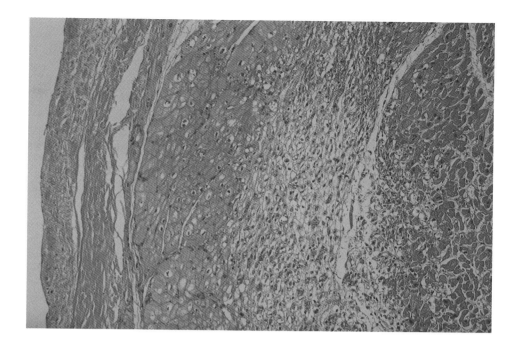

FIG. 339 Histologic findings in the left bundle branch. Granulation tissue can be seen partially involving the left bundle branch. (HE stain, × 90.)

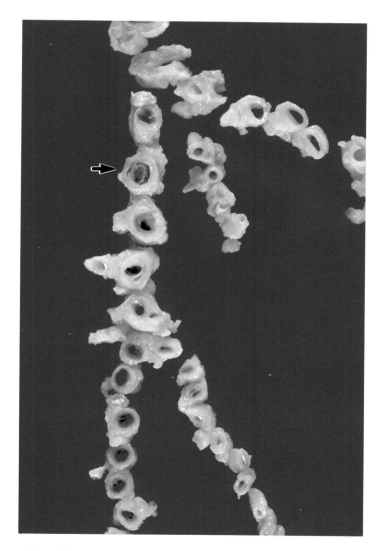

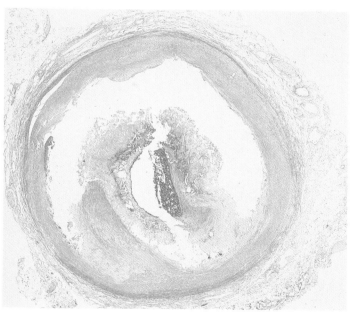

FIG. 341 Histologic findings in the proximal portion of the left anterior descending artery (segment 6). This picture shows the part shown by the arrow in Fig. 340. Complete occlusion by an atheroma and mural thrombus is observed. (HE stain, × 17.5.)

FIG. 340 Left coronary artery. The proximal portion of the left anterior descending artery (segment 6) is completely occluded by thrombi in atheromatous hemorrhages.

CASE 21 ARRHYTHMIA (VENTRICULAR TACHYCARDIA), INFERIOR WALL INFARCTION (6 YEARS)

The patient was a 64-year-old man with both hypertension and diabetes. Six years before death, he was hospitalized for an inferior wall infarct. A pacemaker was implanted because of ventricular tachycardia, atrial fibrillation, and the bradycardia-tachycardia syndrome. Angina pectoris did not occur after the infarction, but the patient was repeatedly hospitalized and discharged because of ventricular tachycardia and heart failure. Left ventriculography

and coronary angiography performed 5 years 8 months before death revealed complete occlusion of segment 3 of the right coronary artery and 99% stenosis of segment 12 of the left circumflex artery. No contraction was evident in the diaphragm surface, the posterior base of the heart, or the posterior wall, and the ejection fraction was 31%. The patient fainted while commuting to work 3 days before death. Resuscitation was successful and he was hospitalized, but ischemic cerebral disturbances ensued, his blood pressure gradually dropped, and he died.

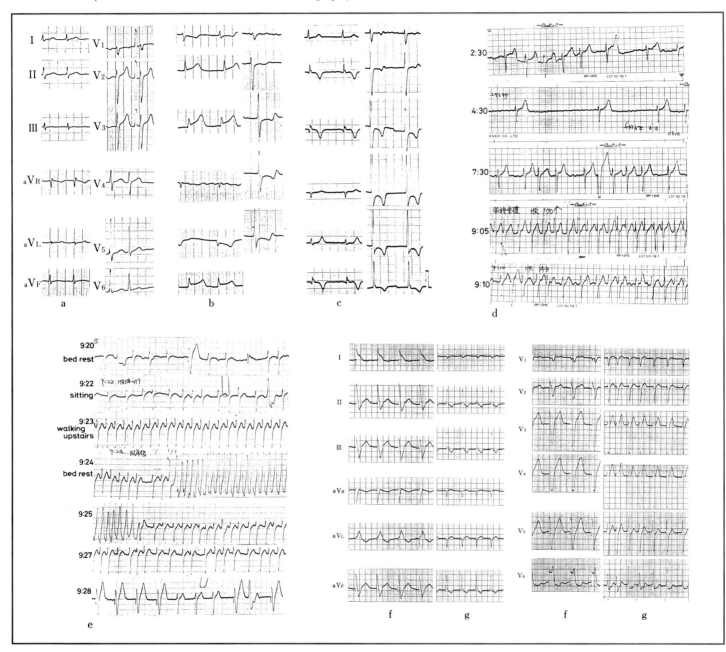

FIG. 342 Electrocardiograms. a: 8 years before death, at onset of infarct; b: 6 years before death, at onset of infarct; c: 6 weeks after b; d: 2 weeks after b, atrial fibrillation and atrioventricular block; e: 5 months after b, atrial fibrillation and ventricular tachycardia; f: 3 days before death, pacemaker rhythm; g: 1 day before, autonomic rhythm.

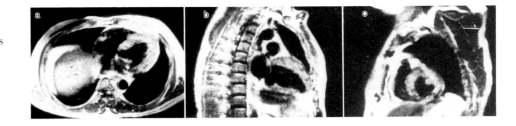

FIG. 343 ECG-synchronized MRI. a: body-axis tomogram; b: long-axis tomogram; c: short-axis tomogram. Thinning of the walls is seen in the short- and long-axis tomograms.

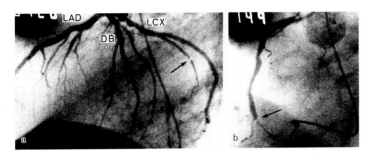

FIG. 344 Coronary angiography a: left coronary artery; b: right coronary artery. (LAD, left anterior descending artery; LCX, left circumflex artery; DB, diagonal branch.)

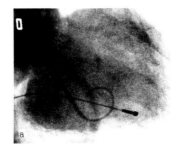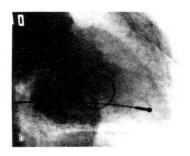

FIG. 345 Left ventriculography. a: end-diastole; b: end-systole.

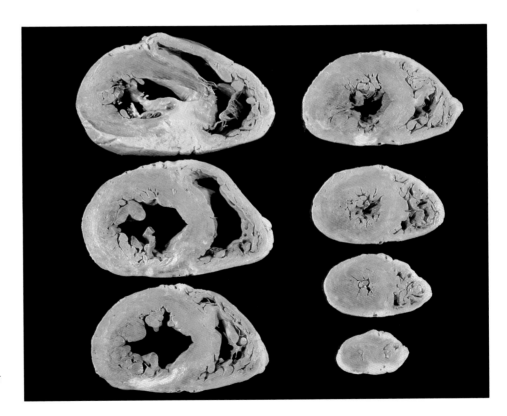

FIG. 346 Transverse sections. Heart weight: 660 g. An old transmural infarction can be seen in the posterior wall of the left ventricle. Discoloration is also present from the anterior to the posterior wall.

Left Ventricular Infarction 137

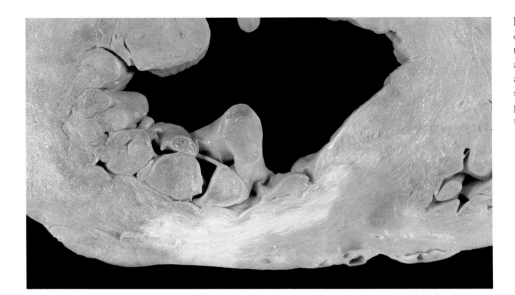

FIG. 347 Transverse section. Close-up view of the myocardial infarction at the level of the center of the papillary muscles. Yellow adipose tissue is seen in an old infarcted area, appearing white. Discoloration can be noted subendocardially from the lateral wall to the posterior portion of the interventricular septum.

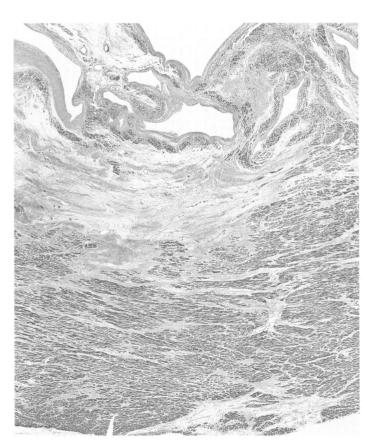

FIG. 348 Histologic findings in the posterior wall of the left ventricle. Fibrosis intermingled with adipose tissue can be seen subendocardially. (Masson trichrome stain, × 9.)

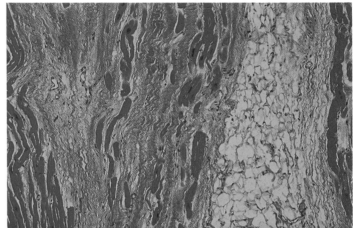

FIG. 349 Histologic findings in the infarcted area. Dense collagen fiber hyperplasia and islands of residual myocardial cells are seen. Fatty infiltration is also present. (HE stain, × 65.)

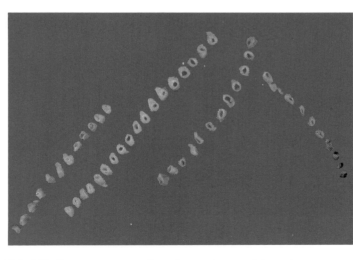

FIG. 350 Coronary arteries. Complete occlusion of the right coronary artery (segment 3) is evident.

Case 22 Epicarditis

The patient was a 65-year-old man who was both hypertensive and diabetic. He was admitted to a local hospital 6 years before death because of an anteroseptal infarction. Heart failure progressed, and the patient changed hospitals after 1 month. Heart failure improved, but fever developed; pericardial friction sounds were heard, and Dressler syndrome was diagnosed. The symptoms were alleviated by administration of a steroid hormone. The left ventricular ejection fraction was 23%. Heart failure persisted after discharge. Six months before death heart failure deteriorated and the patient was readmitted. Thereafter, repeated aggravation and improvement of heart failure occurred. The patient's general condition deteriorated and he died.

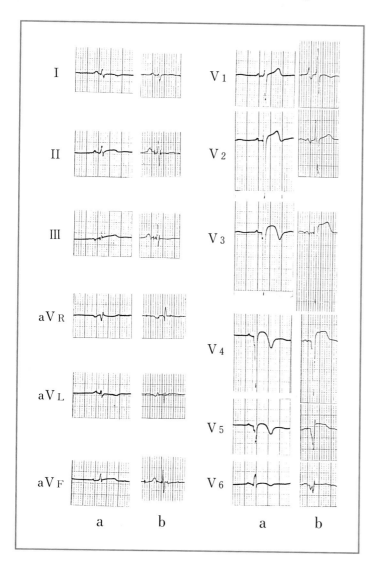

FIG. 351 Electrocardiograms. a: 6 months before death; b: 3 months before death.

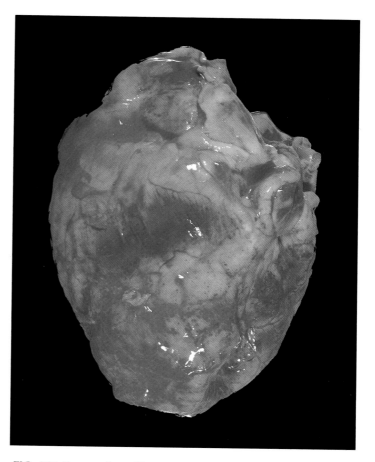

FIG. 352 Front surface of heart. Heart weight: 410 g. Thinning and marked enlargement of the anterolateral wall of the left ventricle are seen. Fibrous epicarditis is present.

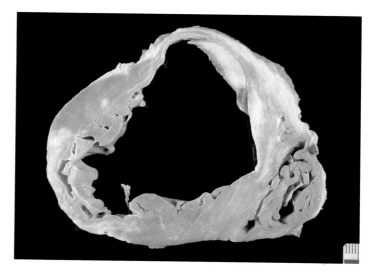

FIG. 353 Transverse section. A white old myocardial infarction can be seen in the anterior wall of the left ventricle and the anterior portion of the interventricular septum. The wall shows thinning and adhesion of a mural thrombus. An old myocardial infarction can also be seen in the posterior wall. The wall shows thinning and aneurysmal enlargement.

6. Right Ventricular Infarction

Right ventricular infarction very rarely occurs alone because of the anatomic distribution of the coronary arteries. It consistently appears concomitantly with posterior wall infarction in the left ventricle. Therefore, right ventricular infarction occurs in the region from the posterior portion of the interventricular septum through the posterior wall of the right ventricle. The advent of new clinical diagnostic techniques in the 1970s, including hemodynamic assessment using Swan-Ganz catheters, two-dimensional echocardiography, and nuclear medicine imaging, enabled the clinical diagnosis of conditions that previously were diagnosed only at autopsy.

Clinically, right ventricular infarction is characterized by (1) comparatively mild signs of pulmonary congestion; (2) a high risk of hypotension, low cardiac output and shock, and a high incidence of arrhythmias, such as severe atrioventricular block; and (3) frequent unresponsiveness of the low cardiac output syndrome and shock to therapy with only catecholamines and diuretics. This disease state differs from that of conventional left ventricular infarction.

Table 9 summarizes the clinical characteristics of right ventricular infarction, and Table 10 summarizes the diagnostic criteria for right ventricular infarction used at the National Cardiovascular Center. In pathologic examinations, right ventricular infarction was noted macroscopically in 14% to 21% and histologically in 34% of all myocardial infarctions. However, clinical diagnosis was possible in only 7% to 13%. In the coronary care unit (CCU) of the National Cardiovascular Center, right ventricular infarction was diagnosed in 9.2% of all acute myocardial infarctions and 29.9% of transmural posterior wall infarctions.

Table 9. Clinical characteristics of right ventricular infarction

1. Physical findings
   Jugular vein dilatation ⎫ Right heart failure sign
   Kussmaul's sign ⎭
   Hypotension ⎫ Sign of low cardiac output
   Oliguria ⎭
2. Electrocardiograms
   Transmural inferior wall infarction
   ST segment elevation in the right chest lead (V_{4R})
   Atrioventricular block
3. Chest x-rays
   Signs of pulmonary congestion image lacking or relatively mild
   Heart shadow enlargement
4. Echocardiography
   Right ventricular chamber enlargement
   Increased end-diastole right/left ventricle inner diameter ratio
   Abnormal right ventricular contraction
   Paradoxical movement of interventricular septum
   Early opening of pulmonary valve

5. Hemodynamics
   Elevated right atrial pressure
   Increased right/left ventricular filling ratio
   Right atrial pressure waveform: deep Y valley (noncompliant pattern)
   Right ventricular pressure waveform: dip and plateau pattern
   Alternating pulse in pulmonary artery
   Low cardiac output
   Drop in right ventricular function curve
6. Nuclear medicine imaging
   ^{99m}Tc pyrophosphate accumulation in right ventricle
   Right ventricular chamber enlargement
   Decreased right ventricular ejection fraction
   Abnormal right ventricular contraction
7. Cardiac angiography
   Lesions in right coronary artery
   Right ventricular enlargement, abnormal contraction

(From Goto Y: Right ventricular infarction, CAD. Nihon Rinsho, Tokyo, 1987, revised from special edition, with permission.)

Table 10. Diagnostic criteria for right ventricular infarction (CCU of National Cardiovascular Center)

A. **Autopsy**
B. **Major criteria**
1. ST segment elevation ($\geq$1 mm) in lead V_{4R}
2. Echocardiograms: no contraction or contraction abnormalities of right ventricle
3. mRA $\geq$10 mmHg and (mPCW-mRA) $\geq$5 mmHg (also possible after volume load)
4. Noncompliant pattern (at least grade 1, also possible after volume load)
5. Pulmonary artery alternating pulse or early rise in pulmonary artery pressure

C. **Minor criteria**
1. Inferior wall infarction
2. Echocardiogram: right ventricular enlargement
3. mRA $\geq$6 mmHg (at rest)
4. Kussmaul's sign (at rest, $\geq$1 mmHg)
5. Accumulation of ^{99m}Tc pyrophosphate in right ventricle

Diagnosis

A. **Postmortem diagnosis**—Presence of right ventricular infarction confirmed at autopsy
B. **Clinical diagnosis**
Definite
1. At least two major criteria
2. One major criterion and at least two minor criteria (however, no overlapping of B-2 and C-2 or B-3 and C-3)
3. At least four minor criteria
Probable
1. One major criterion
2. Three minor criteria

C. **Exclusion criteria**
1. Data for B-3, 4, and 5 and C-2, 3, and 4 are not applicable when constrictive pericarditis or diseases with right ventricular load are present
2. Data for B-3 and 5 and C-3 are not applicable when cardiac tamponade is present

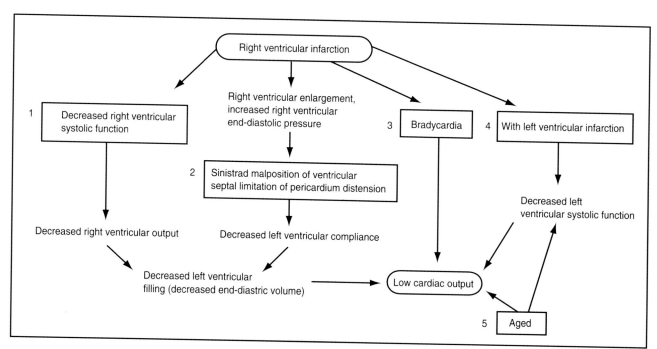

FIG. 354 Mechanism of low cardiac output in right ventricular infarction (From Goto Y: Right ventricular infarction, CAD. Nihon Rinsho, 1987, modified from special edition, with permission.)

CASE 23 RIGHT VENTRICULAR INFARCTION (77 DAYS)

The patient was a 74-year-old man who was hypertensive and diabetic. He developed dyspnea after awakening 77 days before death, and he was admitted to a local hospital. His blood pressure was 70/- mmHg. The ECG indicated atrial fibrillation and type III atrioventricular block; ST segment elevation in leads II, III, and aVF; and ST depression in leads aVL and V_{5-6}. An inferior infarction was diagnosed. He was transferred to the CCU when his shock symptoms did not improve. On admission, his blood pressure was 90/50 mmHg, pulse was 36 beats/min, and SGOT was 2,264 IU/L. Echocardiography revealed no contraction in the inferior and posterior walls of the left ventricle and the posterior wall of the right ventricle. The mean atrial pressure was 7 mmHg (marked Y-shape depression), the mean pulmonary artery wedge pressure was 10 mmHg, and the cardiac index was 2.54 L/min/m² 50 days before death. The low cardiac output syndrome continued. Five days before death, gastrointestinal hemorrhage occurred, and the patient went into shock. Pyothorax developed as a complication, and he died. The maximum CK was 5,430 IU/L and maximum SGOT was 11,000 IU/L.

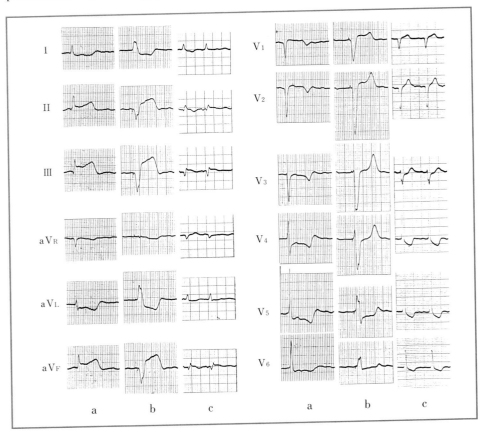

FIG. 355 Electrocardiograms. a: day of onset of infarction, complete atrioventricular block; b: pacemaker rhythm; c: chronic phase.

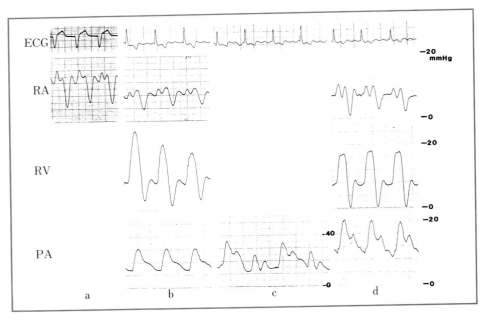

FIG. 356 Intracardiac pressure waveforms of right ventricular infarction. a: 77 days before death; b: 50 days before death; c: 48 days before death, 01:00; d: 48 days before death, 09:50. A deep Y-shaped (noncompliant) pattern in right atrial pressure, a dip and plateau pattern of right ventricular pressure, and alternating pulse of the pulmonary artery are noted. (ECG, electrocardiogram; RA, right atrial pressure; RV, right ventricular pressure; PA, pulmonary artery pressure.)

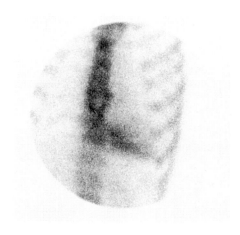

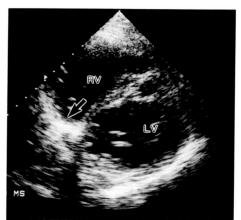

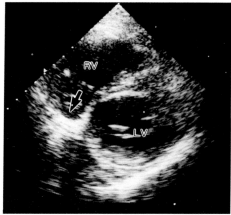

FIG. 357 ^{99m}Tc pyrophosphate myocardial scintigram. Frontal surface aspect. Faint ^{99m}Tc pyrophosphate accumulation is seen in the right ventricle, as well as in the inferoposterior wall.

FIG. 358 Two-dimensional echocardiograms. Thinning and lack of movement (arrows) are seen from within the posterior wall of the left ventricle to the right ventricular wall. The wall thickness of the posterior half of the interventricular septum has decreased. (LV, left ventricle; RV, right ventricle.)

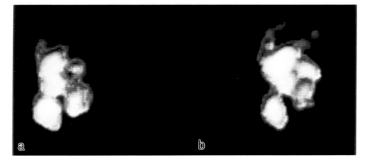

FIG. 359 Gated blood-pool scintigram using ^{99m}Tc-labeled erythrocytes. Left anterior oblique 45° aspect. a: end-diastole; b: end-systole. Enlargement and contraction failure of the right ventricle are evident.

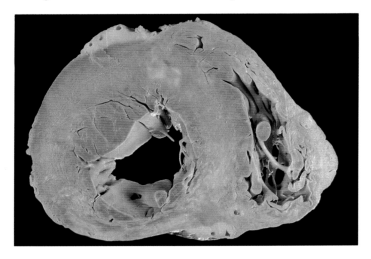

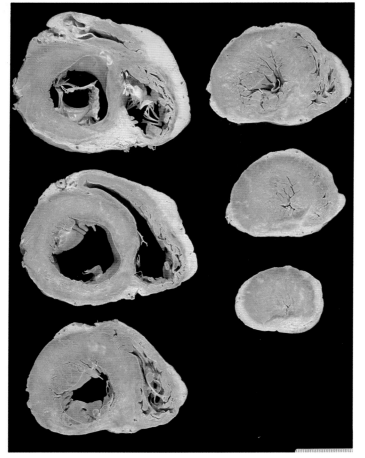

FIG. 360 Transverse section. Level of the center of the papillary muscles. Translucent white fibrosis can be seen in the posterior portion of the interventricular septum, the posterior wall of the left ventricle, and the posterolateral wall of the right ventricle. The posterior wall of the left ventricle shows thinning, and the posteromedial papillary muscles are atrophied.

FIG. 361 Transverse sections. Heart weight: 435 g. Fibrosis is seen in the left ventricle and posterior wall of the right ventricle from the base to the apex of the heart. The posterior wall of the left ventricle is thin and the ventricular chamber is slightly enlarged.

Right Ventricular Infarction 143

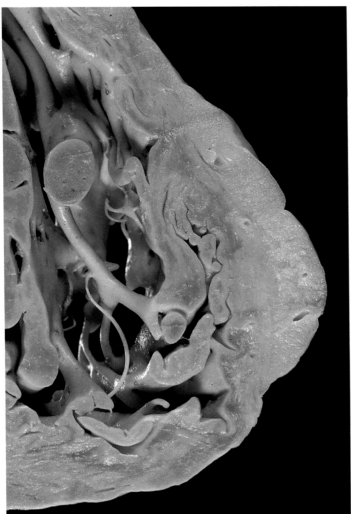

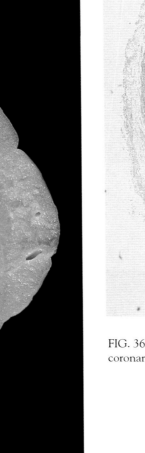

FIG. 364 Histogram of the proximal portion (segment 1) of the right coronary artery. (Masson trichrome stain, × 12.5.)

FIG. 362 Close-up of the infarcted area. The infarcted area in the right ventricle extends almost to the anterior wall.

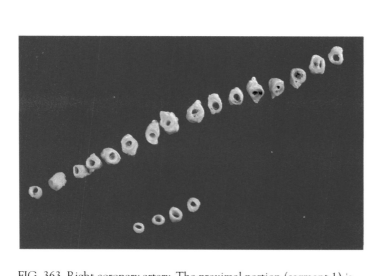

FIG. 363 Right coronary artery. The proximal portion (segment 1) is completely occluded with a hemorrhage into the atheroma.

7. Atrial Infarction

Atrial infarction is a rare disease. There are few characteristic clinical findings, and antemortem diagnosis is difficult. Therefore, the first reports of atrial infarction were derived from autopsy studies. The incidence of atrial infarction has been reported to be 2.8% by Horie et al., 1.7% by Cushing et al., and 7.3% by Wartman et al.

Three ECG changes in atrial infarction are (1) abnormal rhythm in the right atrium, (2) abnormal P waves, and (3) abnormal Ta waves. For (1), atrial fibrillation is the most common type of rhythm abnormality and for (2), some cases may show broad W- or M-shaped nodes or transient high apex. The Ta waves of (3) show low specificity.

Pathologic findings indicate that atrial infarction occurs almost invariably in the right atrium and that it is consistently associated with ventricular infarction.

Anatomically, atrial infarction is reportedly precipitated by severe stenosis and thrombosis of the right coronary artery, occurring proximally to the junction with the sinus node artery. Suspicion of atrial infarction is warranted in patients with stenosis caused by arteriosclerotic plaques at the right coronary artery orifice or aortic dissection extending to the coronary arteries.

In atrial infarction, intra-atrial mural thrombi are frequently encountered and are considered to be the cause of pulmonary thrombotic embolisms in many cases. Atrial rupture is rare.

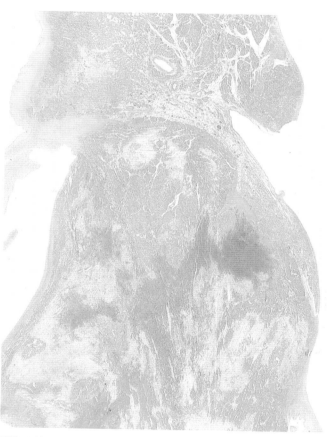

FIG. 365 Atrial infarction case (1). Histologic findings in the interatrial and interventricular septum. An extensive light blue myocardial infarction associated with hemorrhage is seen in the interventricular septum. Light blue fibrosis is also evident in the atrium. (Masson trichrome stain, × 6.)

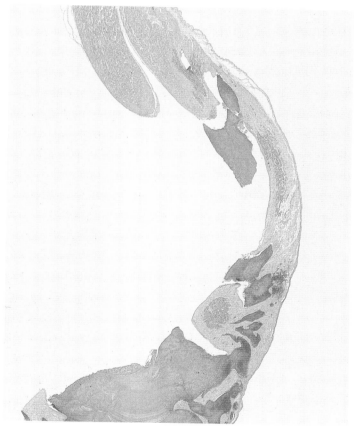

FIG. 366 Atrial infarction case (2). Histologic findings in the right atrium. Sporadic congestion necrosis showing intense eosinophilic staining can be seen in the right atrium. A mural thrombus is present. (HE stain, × 6.)

8. Hemorrhagic Infarction and Reperfusion Injury

Usually, myocardial infarction is pathologically designated as anemic infarction, and the occurrence of hemorrhagic infarction was considered rare. However, the recent increase in the application of cardiovascular surgery, intracoronary thrombolysis (ICT), and percutaneous transluminal coronary angioplasty (PTCA) has provided more opportunities to encounter hemorrhagic infarction at autopsy.

Although a definitive histopathologic definition has yet to be formulated, hemorrhagic infarction can readily be macroscopically distinguished from hemorrhage because the former presents with reddish-brown to black lesions. Histopathologically, hemorrhagic infarction is associated with space-occupying lesions, which are caused by the hemorrhagic lesion pushing away existing myocardial tissue. Therefore, hemorrhagic infarction must be differentiated from simple capillary hyperemia.

Of the approximately 130 autopsies of acute myocardial infarction performed at the National Cardiovascular Center, 6 were considered to involve hemorrhagic infarctions. These included patients with aortic dissection extending to the coronary artery orifice, coronary bypass grafting, and left ventricular assist devices.

Even when the time of reperfusion is uncertain, some cases lacking pathologic evidence of coronary artery thrombosis, but showing peripheral thrombus fragments, may have undergone embolism. Pathologically, therefore, reperfusion can be presumed to have occurred.

In all cases, hemorrhagic foci were localized to within the area of infarction, and the myocardial lesions seen within the hemorrhagic foci were diverse. The most commonly noted change was the persistence of coagulation necrosis in a frozen state, indicating a significant delay in the healing process. In infarcted areas other than hemorrhagic foci, changes expressing the normal evolution of infarction were noted.

CASE 24 HEMORRHAGIC INFARCTION

The patient was a 71-year-old man who smoked 40 cigarettes a day. He did not have hypertension or diabetes. An anterior wall infarction had occurred 4.5 years before. Thereafter, exertional angina pectoris continued, and 77 days before death he was admitted to the coronary care unit (CCU) for unstable angina pectoris. Left ventriculography and coronary angiography revealed 90% stenosis of segment 1 and complete occlusion of segment 6 of the right coronary artery. No contraction was noted at the apex. Weakened contraction was seen at the diaphragm surface and posterior basal, septal, and posterior walls. The ejection fraction was 45%. Because of resistance to conservative therapy, he underwent coronary bypass grafting (segment 4 of the right coronary artery, first diagonal branch) 9 days before death. A fever appeared on the third postoperative day; the patient developed sepsis and died.

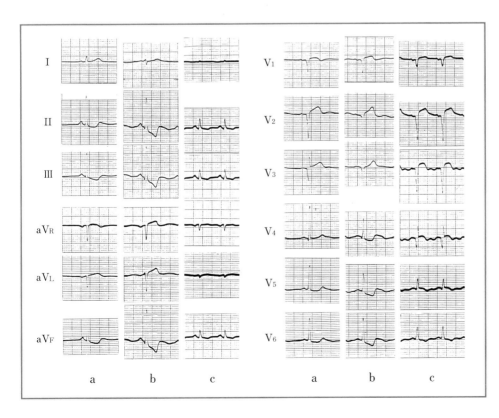

FIG. 367 Electrocardiograms. a: 13 days before death, control; b: 9 days before death, during chest pains; c: 7 days before death, postoperatively.

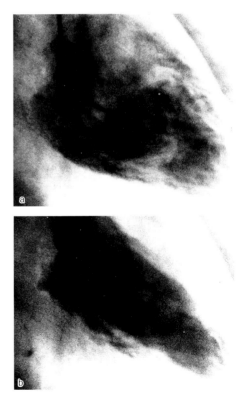

FIG. 368 Left ventriculography. a: end-diastole; b: end-systole.

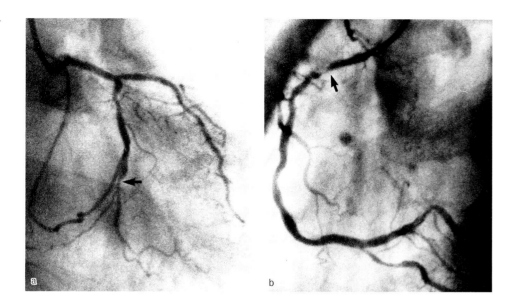

FIG. 369 Coronary angiography. a: left coronary artery; b: right coronary artery. The left anterior descending artery is completely occluded.

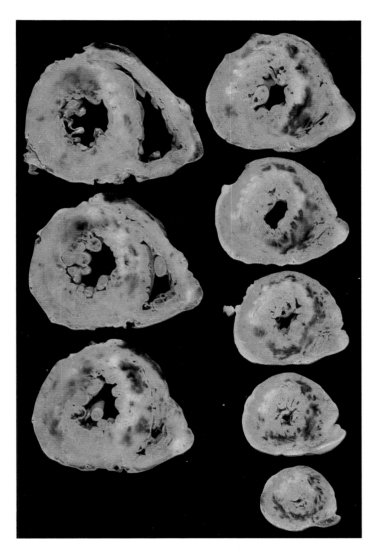

FIG. 370 Transverse sections. Heart weight 440 g. White fibrosis is seen mainly subendocardially in the anterolateral wall of the left ventricle and the anterior portion of the interventricular septum from the level of the tendinous cords to the apex. Discoloration associated with hemorrhage can be seen around the old infarction, in the posterior wall of the left ventricle, and in the interventricular septum.

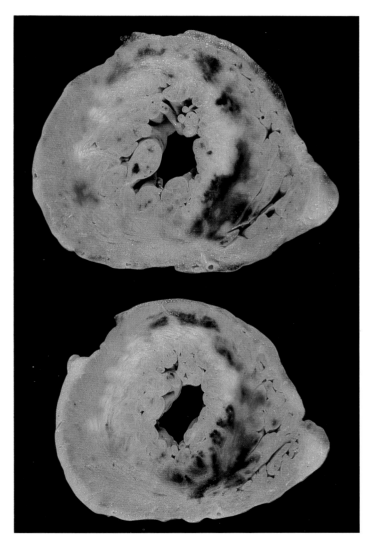

FIG. 371 Transverse sections. Areas of translucent white fibrosis are seen mainly subendocardially in the anterolateral wall of the left ventricle and the anterior portion of the interventricular septum. Hemorrhagic infarction is present around the old infarction and in the posterior portion of the interventricular septum.

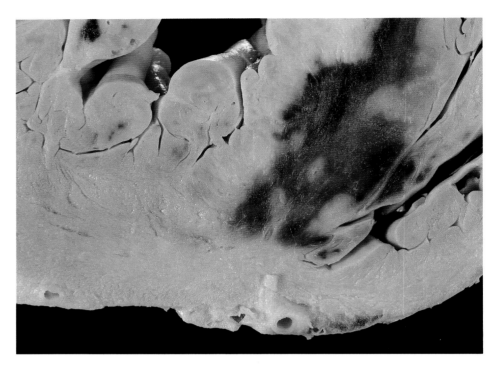

FIG. 372 Close-up view of the infarcted area. Translucent white fibrosis is seen subendocardially, and discoloration associated with marked hemorrhage is seen inside the fibrous area.

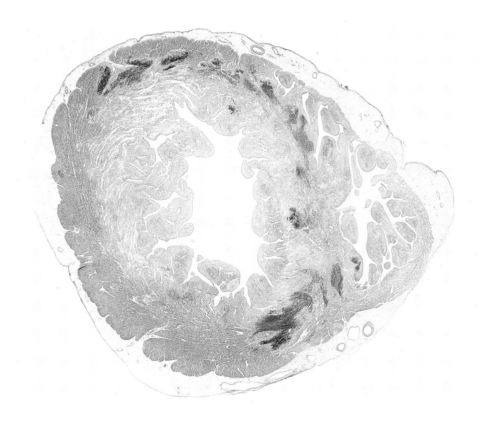

FIG. 373 Histologic transverse section. Fibrosis extending throughout almost the entire circumference can be seen subendocardially in the left ventricle. Reddish-violet hemorrhagic foci are present in the anterior wall, interventricular septum, and posterior wall. (Masson trichrome stain.)

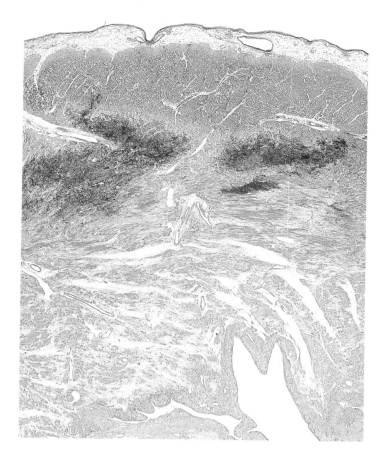

FIG. 374 Histologic findings in the left ventricular anterior wall. Fibrosis can be seen subendocardially, bordered by reddish-violet hemorrhagic infarction. (Masson trichrome stain, × 8.)

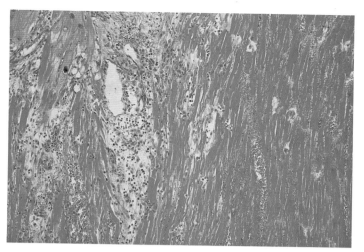

FIG. 375 Histologic findings in the infarcted area. The myocardial fibers are eosinophilic, the striations have disappeared, and cells have become denucleated. Infiltration with numerous inflammatory cells is seen interstitially. Marked hemorrhage is also present. (HE stain, × 65.)

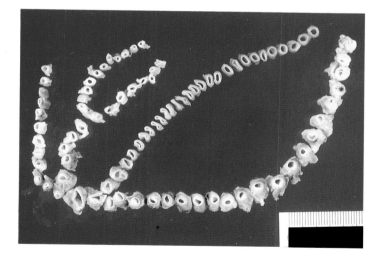

FIG. 376 Right coronary artery. Severe stenosis of more than 90% can be seen in the proximal part. The great saphenous vein bypass is patent.

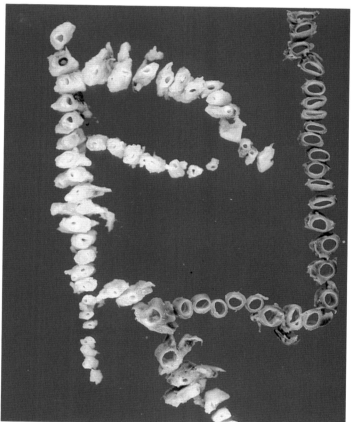

FIG. 377 Left coronary artery. The main trunk is completely occluded by an atheroma. The left anterior descending artery is almost completely occluded at the junction of the first diagonal branch, but the left circumflex artery shows less than 50% stenosis. The bypass to the left anterior descending artery is patent.

CASE 25 HEMORRHAGIC INFARCTION (41 DAYS)

The patient was a 64-year-old man who smoked 30 cigarettes a day and was not hypertensive or diabetic. Dyspnea occurred at 00:10, 41 days before death. He was examined by a local physician at 13:00 because of chest pains, cold sweat, and vomiting. He was transferred to the CCU because of repeated episodes of ventricular fibrillation. On admission, his blood pressure was 60/-mmHg, CK 403 IU/L, and SGOT 80 IU/L. On the ECG, ST segment depression was noted in leads II, III, aVF, and V_{1-2} and ST

segment elevation in leads I, aVL, and V_{3-6}. Coronary angiography revealed 75% stenosis of segment 5 of the left coronary artery and 50% stenosis of segment 6 of the left anterior descending artery. ICT was performed, but the degree of stenosis remained unchanged. Coronary bypass grafting (segment 7 of the left anterior descending artery and segment 14 of the posterolateral branch) was performed, and a left ventricular assist device was inserted. Postoperatively, the patient became dependent on the assist device, multiple organ failure occurred, and he died.

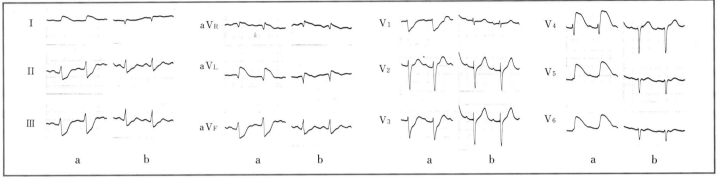

FIG. 378 Electrocardiograms. a: 41 days before death, 4 hours after onset of infarction; b: postoperatively.

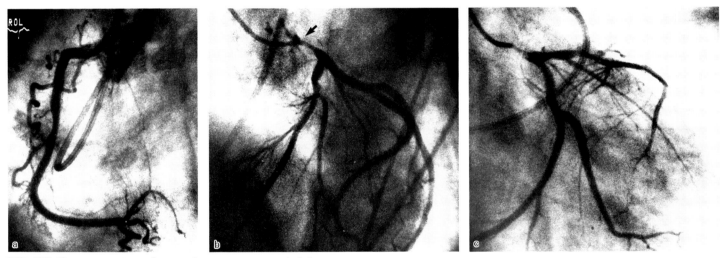

FIG. 379 Coronary angiography. a: right coronary artery; b: left coronary artery; c: left coronary artery after intracoronary injection of 480,000 units of urokinase.

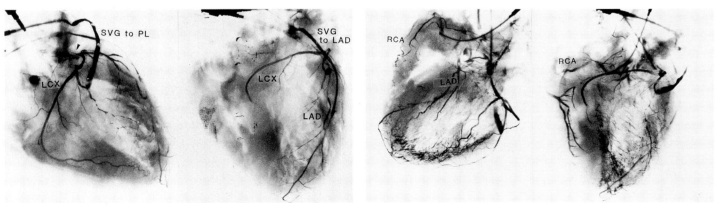

FIG. 380 Postmortem angiography. (LAD, left anterior descending artery; LCX, left circumflex artery; RCA, right coronary artery; SVG to LAD, saphenous vein graft to left anterior descending artery; SVG to PL, saphenous vein graft to posterolateral branch.)

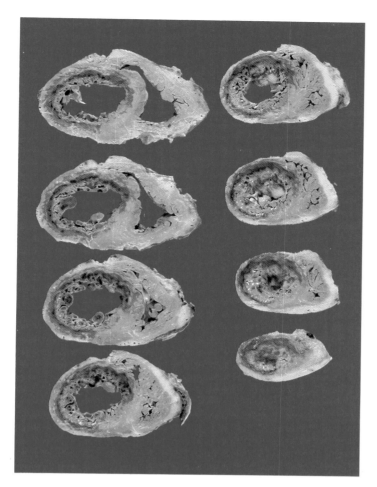

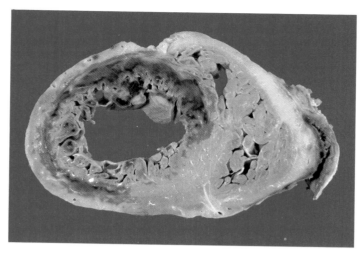

FIG. 382 Transverse section. Level about one-third the distance from the apex. A hemorrhagic infarction can be seen in part of the antero-lateral and posterior walls of the left ventricle and the anterior portion of the interventricular septum. Mural thrombi are present.

FIG. 381 Transverse sections. Heart weight: 470 g. A transmural infarction associated with hemorrhage extends throughout almost the entire circumference of the left ventricle from the level of the tendinous cords to the apex. Only part of the posterior portion of the interventricular septum and posterior wall of the left ventricle remain unaffected. The ventricular chamber is enlarged, and a thrombus is present in the apex.

FIG. 383 Close-up view of the infarcted area. Infarction associated with hemorrhage is seen subendocardially. Laterally, the infarcted area is translucent and slightly concave. Several layers of myocardium remain directly under the endocardium.

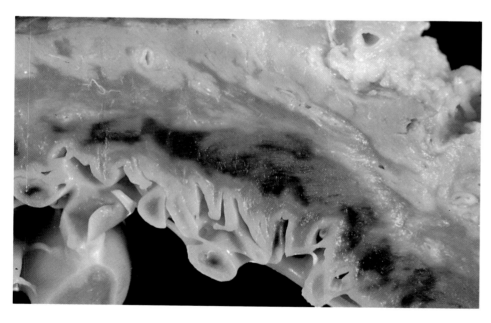

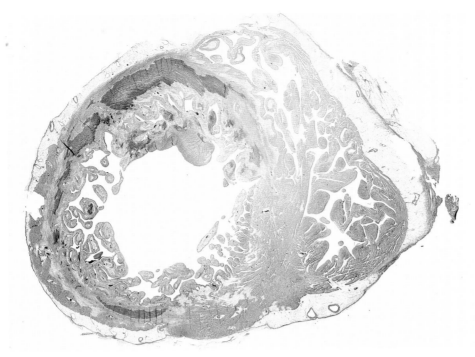

FIG. 384 Histologic transverse section. Extensive fibrosis can be seen in the anterior portion of the interventricular septum and anterolateral wall, extending to the posterior wall of the left ventricle. The center of the fibrous region, stained reddish-violet, is coagulation necrosis associated with hemorrhage. (Masson trichrome stain.)

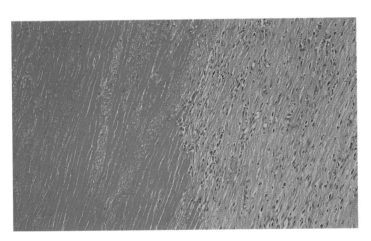

FIG. 385 Histologic findings in the infarcted area. Many fibroblasts, sparse collagen fibers, and fibrosis including cells containing hemosiderin are present. Coagulation necrosis is still seen in sites of marked hemorrhage, indicating delayed healing. (HE stain, × 65.)

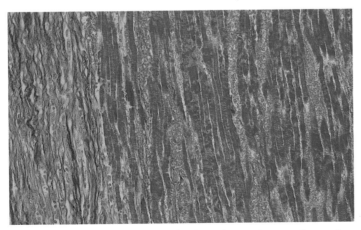

FIG. 386 Histologic findings in the infarcted area. A striated muscular structure exhibiting supercontraction is still seen in the coagulation necrosis located at the site of hemorrhagic infarction. (Masson trichrome stain, × 130.)

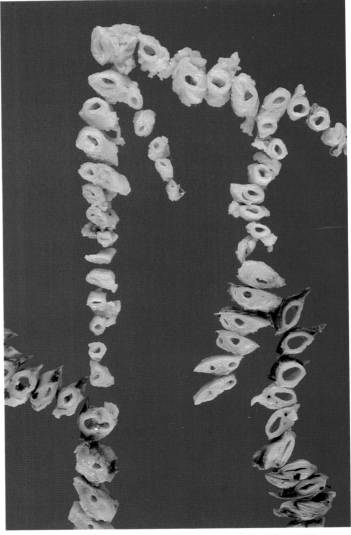

FIG. 387 Left coronary artery. Severe stenosis of more than 75% is seen in the proximal part of the left anterior descending artery. The great saphenous vein bypass to the left anterior descending artery and acute marginal branch is patent.

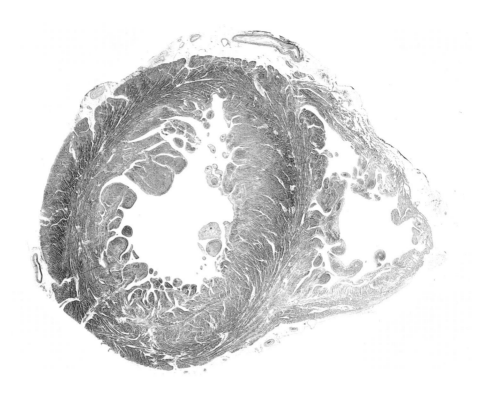

FIG. 396 Histologic transverse section. A darkly stained area is seen subendocardially in the anterior portion of the interventricular septum and anterolateral wall of the left ventricle. (Masson trichrome stain.)

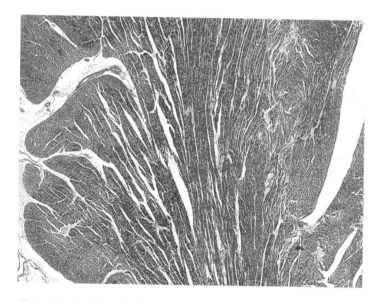

FIG. 397 Histologic findings in the anterior wall of the left ventricle. An area of marked contraction band necrosis is noted subendocardially. (Masson trichrome stain, × 7.5.)

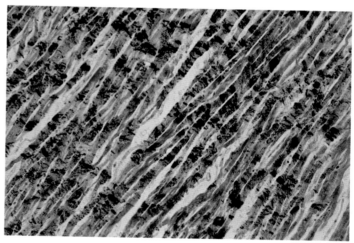

FIG. 398 Histologic findings in the infarcted area. The myocardial fibers are dissociated and marked contraction band necrosis is seen. (Heidenhain's iron and HE stain, × 130.)

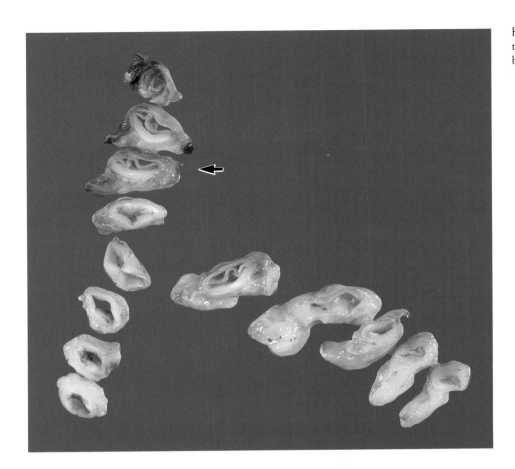

FIG. 399 Left coronary artery. The main trunk and left circumflex artery appear double-barreled because of the dissection.

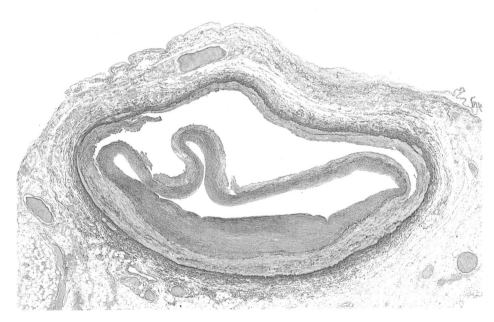

FIG. 400 Histologic findings in the left main trunk. The part designated by the arrow in Fig. 399. Dissection of the media can be noted over half the circumference. Fibrous thickening is evident in the intima. (Elastica van Gieson stain, × 18.5.)

Case 27 Diabetes

The patient was a 67-year-old woman who was hypertensive and diabetic. Exertional angina pectoris appeared 1 year 4 months before death. She was hospitalized for unstable angina pectoris 4 months later, and an inferior wall infarction of Killip I and Forrester I occurred during hospitalization. The maximum serum CK was 8,195 IU/L. Left ventriculography and coronary angiography taken 10 months before death revealed 99% stenosis of segment 1 of the right coronary artery, 90% stenosis of segment 7 of the left anterior descending artery, and 75% stenosis of segment 11 and complete occlusion of segment 12 of the left circumflex artery. No contraction was found in the apex, diaphragm, or posterior basal or septal walls. The ejection fraction was 29%. Rehabilitation was carried out gradually. Seven months before death a nontransmural anterior wall infarction of Killip II and Forrester II occurred. The serum CK was 595 IU/L. Thereafter, treatment of heart failure became difficult, and repeated aggravation and improvement developed. Three days before death, fever developed followed by renal dysfunction leading to death.

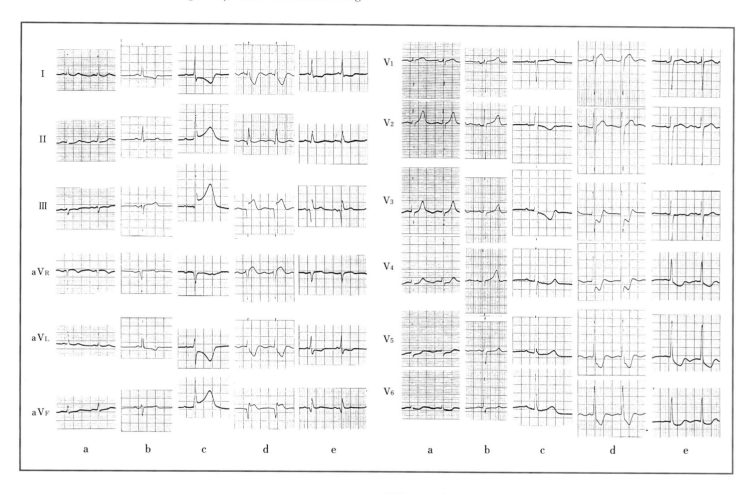

FIG. 401 Electrocardiograms. a: 1 year before death at onset of chest pain; b: at rest; c: onset of inferior wall infarct; d: 11 months before death, during chest pain; e: 26 days before death, at rest.

FIG. 402 Myocardial scintigrams. a: frontal aspect; b: left anterior oblique 45° aspect; c: left lateral aspect. A defect image corresponding to the inferoposterior wall is noted.

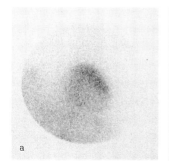
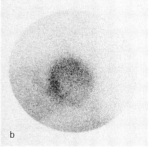
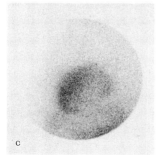

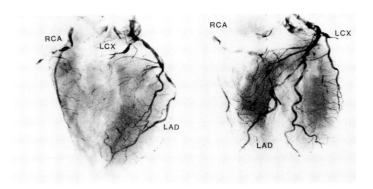

FIG. 403 Postmortem angiography. (LAD, left anterior descending artery; LCX, left circumflex artery; RCA, right coronary artery.)

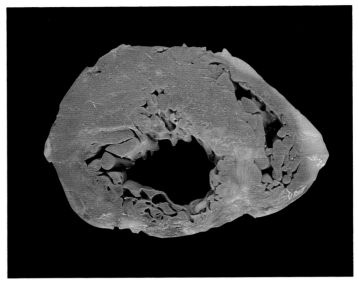

FIG. 405 Transverse section. Level of the center of the papillary muscles. Translucent fibrosis can be seen in the posteromedial wall of the left ventricle, and white, partially translucent fibrosis is present in the posterior portion of the interventricular septum. The posterior wall is thin and the posteromedial papillary muscles are atrophied.

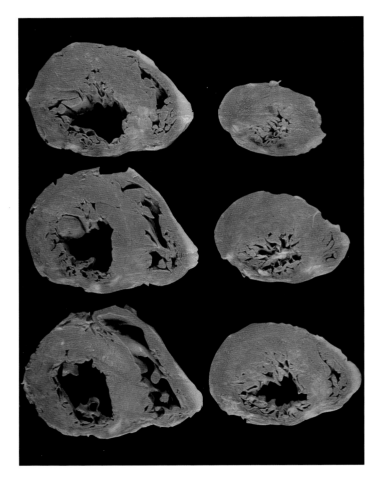

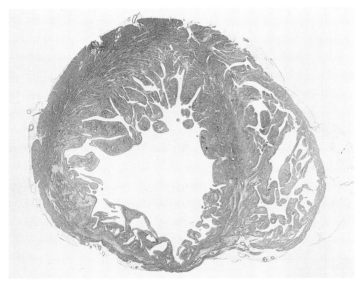

FIG. 406 Histologic transverse section. An old myocardial infarction is seen in the posterior portion of the interventricular septum and posterior wall of the left ventricle. Many areas of sporadic fibrosis are noted subendocardially. (Masson trichrome stain.)

FIG. 404 Transverse sections. Heart weight: 370 g. An old white translucent transmural infarction is seen in the posterolateral wall of the left ventricle and the posterior portion of the interventricular septum from the level of the tendinous cords through the apex. The posterior wall is thin and the posteromedial papillary muscles are atrophied.

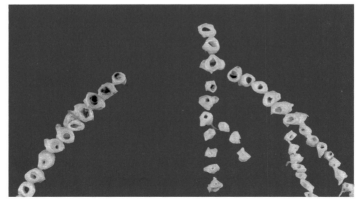

FIG. 407 Coronary arteries. Severe atheromatous stenosis is present in the proximal parts of the right coronary artery, left anterior descending artery, and left circumflex artery.

CASE 28 HYPERCHOLESTEROLEMIA

The patient was a 48-year-old man who was not hypertensive or diabetic. Acute myocardial infarction occurred 12 years and 1 year before death. Thereafter, he often experienced chest pains on effort. Symptoms of heart failure developed 36 days before death, and he was hospitalized. The heart failure was improved by treatment with diuretic and nitrate preparations.

On gated blood-pool scintigraphy, the ejection fraction was 35%. Chest pains appeared 13 hours before death. In the ECG, ST segment depression was seen in leads V_{5-6}. Dyspnea became worse and cardiogenic shock occurred. The patient suffered repeated episodes of ventricular tachycardia and ventricular fibrillation, resulting in death.

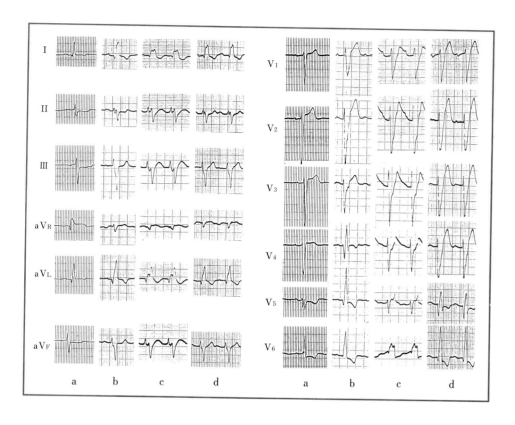

FIG. 408 Electrocardiograms. a: 1 year before death; b: 36 days before death, at admission; c: 24 days before death, at rest, d: 13 hours before death.

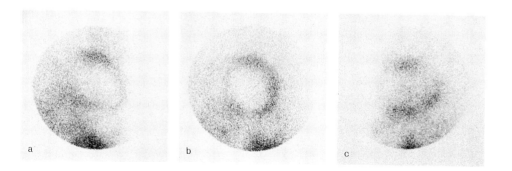

FIG. 409 Myocardial scintigrams. a: frontal aspect; b: left anterior oblique 45° aspect; c: lateral aspect. The heart chamber is enlarged, and the uptake of thallium by the myocardium is speckled. Extensive defect images are seen from the anterolateral wall to the apex, and lesions are suspected in three branches.

Miscellaneous Myocardial Infarction   161

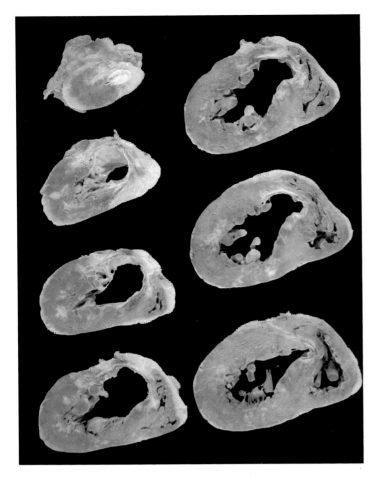

FIG. 410 Transverse sections. Heart weight: 550 g. An old transmural infarction can be seen in the anterior portion of the interventricular septum and anterior wall of the left ventricle from the level of the tendinous cords to the apex. The walls are thin, and the ventricular chamber shows aneurysmal enlargement. Small areas of fibrosis are evident sporadically in the lateral and posterior walls.

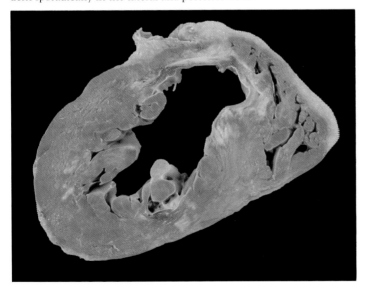

FIG. 411 Transverse section. Level of the center of the papillary muscles. An old white transmural infarction is seen in the anterior portion of the interventricular septum and anterior walls of the left ventricle. The walls are thin and the ventricular chamber shows mass-like enlargement. Small areas of fibrosis are also evident in the lateral and posterior walls.

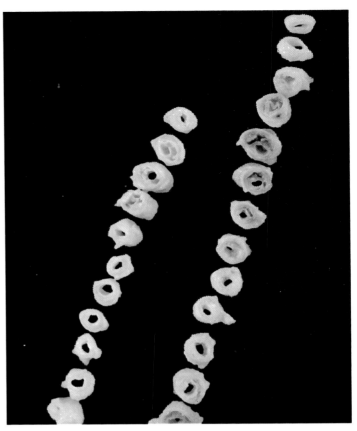

FIG. 412 Right coronary artery. Atheromatous stenosis of more than 75% can be seen in the proximal and distal portions.

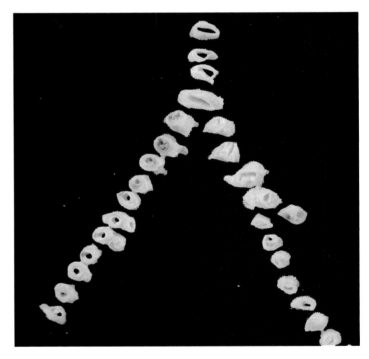

FIG. 413 Left coronary artery. Severe atheromatous stenosis of more than 90% can be seen in the proximal part of the left anterior descending artery. The left circumflex artery shows stenosis of more than 75%.

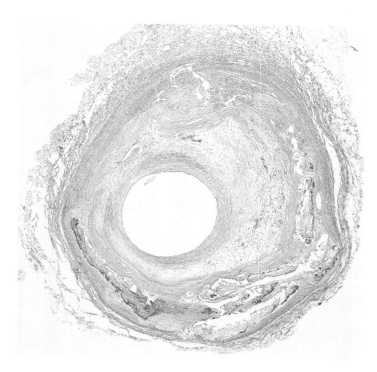

FIG. 414 Histologic findings in the left anterior descending artery. (Masson trichrome stain, × 23.)

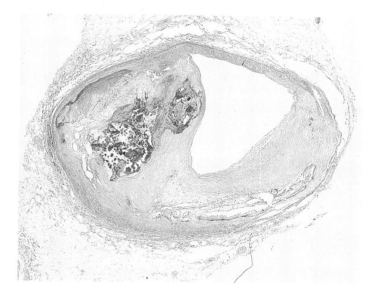

FIG. 415 Histologic findings in the left circumflex artery. (Masson trichrome stain, × 15.5.)

CASE 29 KAWASAKI DISEASE

The patient was a 1-year, 8-month-old girl. At 8 months of age, she developed Kawasaki disease with all six of the main symptoms. At 13 months, left ventriculography and coronary angiography revealed aneurysms in the right and left coronary arteries. Seven days before death, she suddenly felt bad and her face grew pale. Six days before death, she was admitted to the hospital. In the ECG, ST segment depression was seen in leads V_{5-6}. After admission, ST segment depression was seen when she cried or was very active. One day before death, marked ST segment depression and negative T waves were seen in leads II, III, aVF, and V_{3-6}. The serum CK was 225 IU/L. Ten hours before death chest pains appeared. ST segment changes were the same and the serum CK was 182 IU/L. Thereafter, bradycardia developed, her blood pressure dropped, and she died.

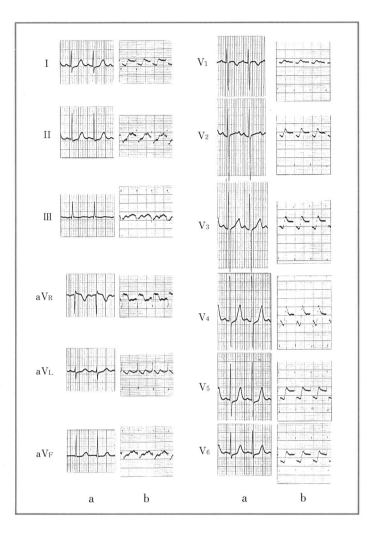

FIG. 416 Electrocardiograms. a: 8 days before death, control; b: 2 days before death, during chest pains.

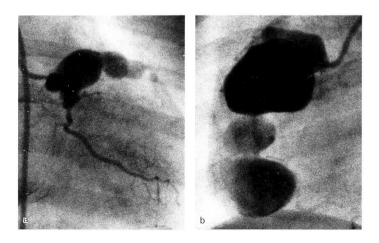

FIG. 417 Coronary angiography. a: left coronary artery; b: right coronary artery.

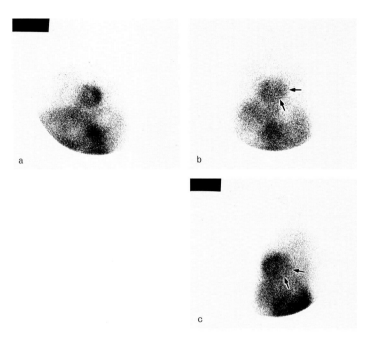

FIG. 418 Myocardial scintigrams. a: frontal aspect; b: left anterior oblique 45° aspect, position; c: left lateral aspect. Defect and reduction are seen from the inferoposterior wall to the lateral wall.

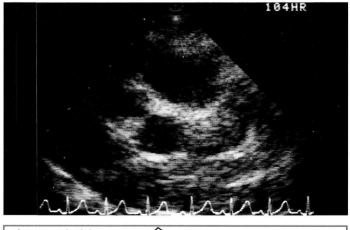

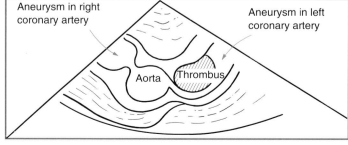

FIG. 419 Two-dimensional echocardiograms. Aneurysms are present in the left and right coronary arteries. Thrombosis is noted in the left coronary artery aneurysm.

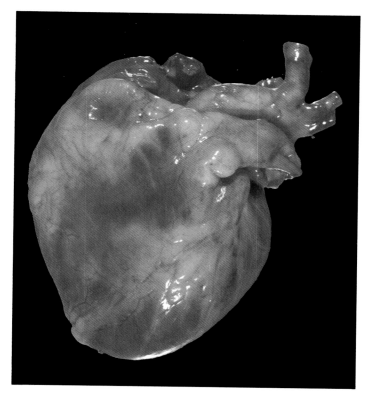

FIG. 420 Front surface of the heart. Marked aneurysmal enlargement is present in the right coronary artery and the proximal part of the left anterior descending artery.

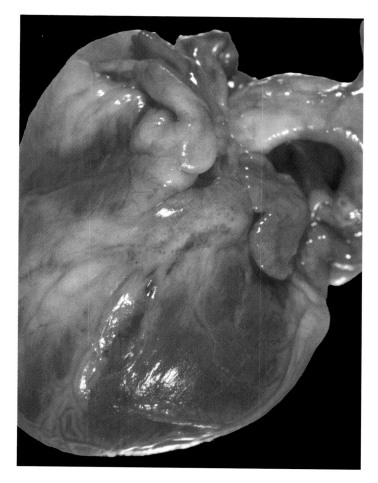

FIG. 421 Aneurysm of the left anterior descending artery. The left anterior descending artery shows marked aneurysmal enlargement from the origin.

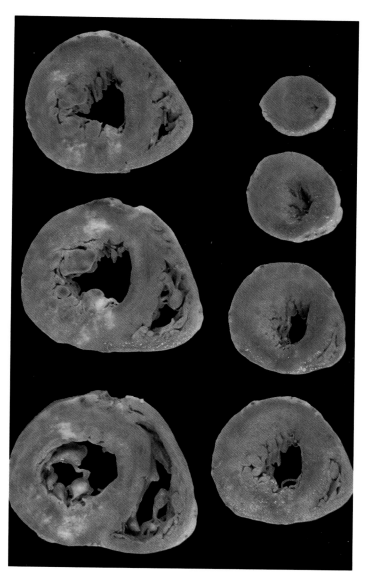

FIG. 422 Transverse sections. Discoloration is seen in the anterolateral wall of the left ventricle and the anterior portion of the interventricular septum from the level of the tendinous cords to the apex. Small areas of fibrosis are observed sporadically.

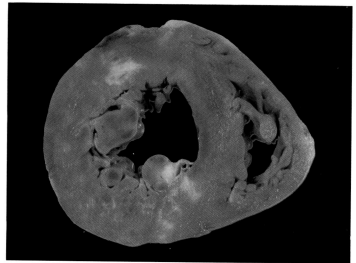

FIG. 423 Transverse section. Level of the center of the papillary muscles. Discoloration is evident in the anterolateral wall of the left ventricle and anterior portion of the interventricular septum. Small areas of fibrosis are seen in the anterior and posterior walls of the left ventricle and the posteromedial papillary muscles.

Miscellaneous Myocardial Infarction   165

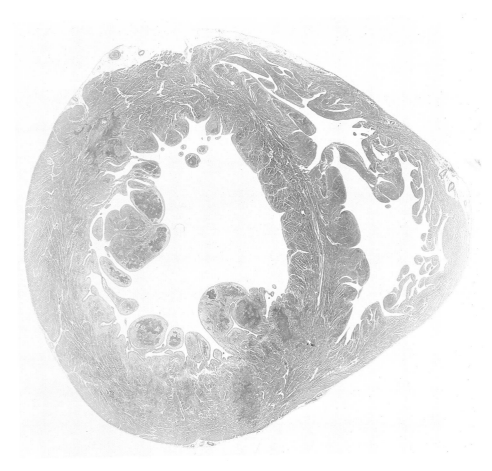

FIG. 424 Histologic transverse section. Fibrosis is noted in the anterior and posterior walls of the left ventricle. (Masson trichrome stain.)

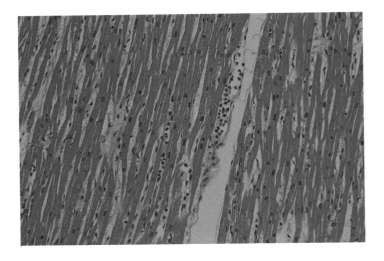

FIG. 425 Histologic findings in the infarcted area. Myocardial fibers are dissociated because of interstitial edema. Neutrophil margination is observed in the capillaries. (HE stain, × 130.)

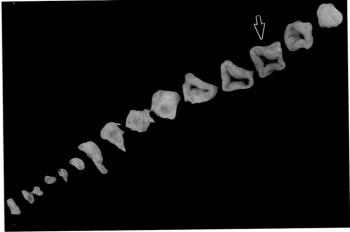

FIG. 426 Right coronary artery. A spindle-shaped aneurysm is seen from the proximal portion. Fibrous thickening is present inside the artery, and severe stenosis is evident at the end of the aneurysm.

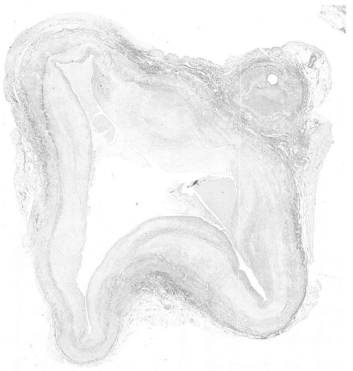

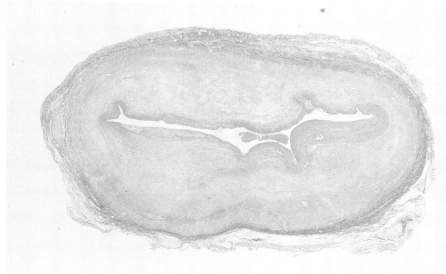

FIG. 427 Histologic findings in the right coronary artery (the part designated by the arrow in Fig. 426). The medium has almost completely disappeared and a large aneurysm has formed. The intima shows fibrous thickening and thrombus adhesion. Aneurysmal enlargement is present in the branches, and marked stenosis has occurred as a result of intimal hypertrophy. (Elastica van Gieson stain, × 7.)

FIG. 428 Left coronary artery. A marked aneurysm is present from the origin of the left anterior descending artery, and fibrous hypertrophy is seen inside the artery. The left circumflex artery shows hypoplasia.

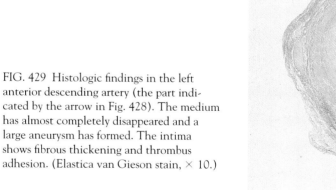

FIG. 429 Histologic findings in the left anterior descending artery (the part indicated by the arrow in Fig. 428). The medium has almost completely disappeared and a large aneurysm has formed. The intima shows fibrous thickening and thrombus adhesion. (Elastica van Gieson stain, × 10.)

10. Percutaneous Transluminal Coronary Angioplasty and Intracoronary Thrombolysis

The major problem with PTCA is a high incidence of restenosis, which usually occurs in 30% to 50% of patients. The mechanism causing restenosis appears to involve thrombosis and smooth muscle cell proliferation in the dilated area. Factors conducive to restenosis include severe coronary spasm, insufficient dilation, with initial dilation being less than 50%, hardening of the wall due to calcification, and multibranch lesions, but many factors remain unclear.

The recent introduction of percutaneous transluminal coronary angioplasty (PTCA) and intracoronary thrombolysis (ICT) has contributed significantly to the treatment of patients with ischemic heart disease.

ICT is a therapeutic technique for the lysis of intracoronary thrombi associated with acute myocardial infarction or an occasional patient with refractory unstable angina pectoris (Fig. 431).

The principal objective of PTCA is to dilate organic stenosis of the coronary arteries. Currently, the range of indications for PTCA is being broadened, based on additional clinical experience, greater technical expertise, and improved equipment. PTCA is now indicated for at least some of the following difficult-to-manage lesions and conditions: (1) multibranch lesions, (2) calcified blood vessels, (3) eccentric stenosis, (4) long stenosed vessels, (5) junctional stenosis, (6) completely occluded vessels, (7) elderly patients, (8) acute myocardial infarction, (9) reduced left ventricular function, and (10) after coronary bypass grafting (Figs. 432 to 435).

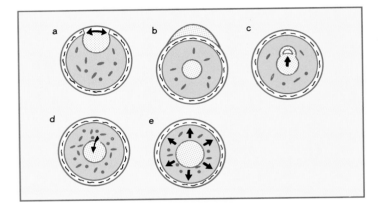

FIG. 430 Mechanism of luminal diameter expansion by PTCA. a: fissure in the intima and media. When the lumen is eccentric, fissures tend to occur more in healthy areas on the opposite side than in areas with atheromas; b: dissection of the media; c: dissociation of the intima. Peripheral embolism might occur because of dissociation. The lumen at the site of dissociation is slightly enlarged; d: release of atheroma into the lumen; e: compression of the atheroma. This is currently considered to be improbable. (From Horimoto S: Mechanisms of luminal diameter expansion by PTCA. Byori to Rinsho :4, 1986, with permission.)

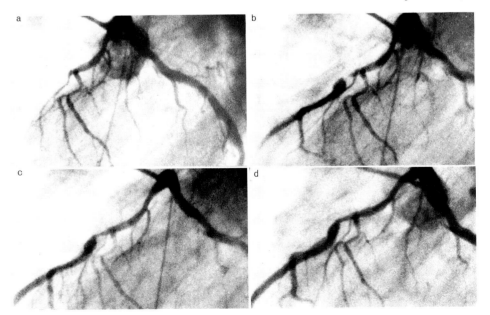

FIG. 431 ICT of acute myocardial infarction. a: control angiography of left coronary artery; b: after intracoronary injection of 480,000 units of urokinase; c: after intracoronary injection of 720,000 units of urokinase; d: after 1 month. Case treated 2 hours after onset of anterior wall infarction.

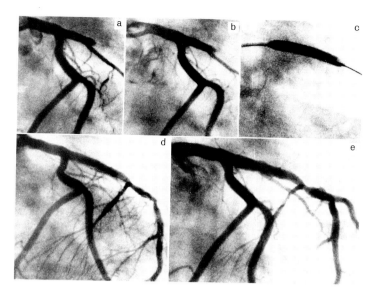

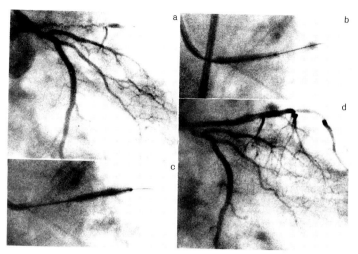

FIG. 432 ICT and PTCA of acute myocardial infarction. a: control angiography of left coronary artery; b: after intracoronary injection of 960,000 units of urokinase; c: during PTCA; d: after PTCA; e: after 3 weeks. Case treated 4 hours after onset of anterior wall infarction. Because recanalization of the left anterior descending artery was not achieved by ICT, PTCA was performed.

FIG. 433 PTCA of a long stenotic lesion. a: control; b,c: during PTCA; d: after PTCA. The lesion was 31 mm long from the proximal part of the left anterior descending artery to the junction of a large septal branch.

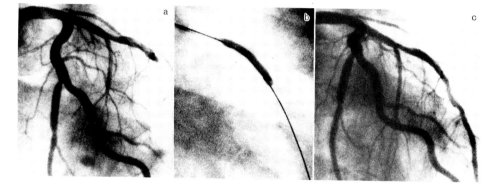

FIG. 434 PTCA of a chronic completely occluded lesion. a: control; b: during PTCA; c: after PTCA.

FIG. 435 PTCA of a stenotic lesion at a bifurcation. a: control; b: PTCA in anterior descending artery; c: PTCA in diagonal branch; d: after PTCA. PTCA was performed on a stenotic lesion at the bifurcation of the anterior descending artery and diagonal branch. Guide-wires were passed through both vessels to prevent one vessel from being occluded while the other one was being dilated.

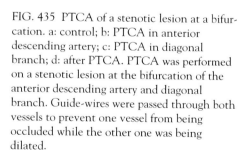

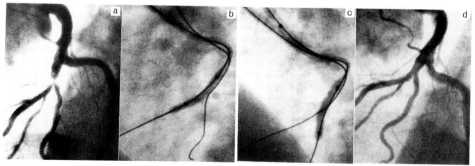

Case 30 PTCA (1)

The patient was a 77-year-old woman who was hypertensive and diabetic. At about 7 PM, 57 days before death, chest pain occurred and continued for 30 to 40 minutes. The patient was admitted to the coronary care unit (CCU) with a diagnosis of an inferoposterior wall infarction 54 days before death. On admission, her blood pressure was 124/72 mmHg, pulse rate was 84 beats/min and regular, CK 645 IU/L, and SGOT 174 IU/L. On the electrocardiogram (ECG), ST segment elevation was noted in leads I, II, aV$_F$, and V$_6$. R wave height elevation in lead V$_{S1-2}$, and R wave height depression in lead V$_5$ were observed. The mean pulmonary artery wedge pressure was 10 mmHg, and the cardiac index was 2.10 L/min/m^2. The infarction was Killip type I and Forrester type III. Left ventriculography and coronary angiography were performed for ICT 52 days before death. Complete occlusion of segment 14 of the left circumflex artery was observed. On left ventriculography, no contraction was present in the apex, diaphragm surface, or posterior wall. The ejection fraction was 40% and mitral insufficiency was moderately severe. ICT was unsuccessful. Frequent episodes of chest pain occurred beginning 33 days before death, and PTCA was performed 25 days before death. The stenosis of segment 14 of the left circumflex artery was improved to 50%. Thereafter, chest pain disappeared, but pneumonia and gastrointestinal bleeding occurred. Her general condition worsened, and the patient died.

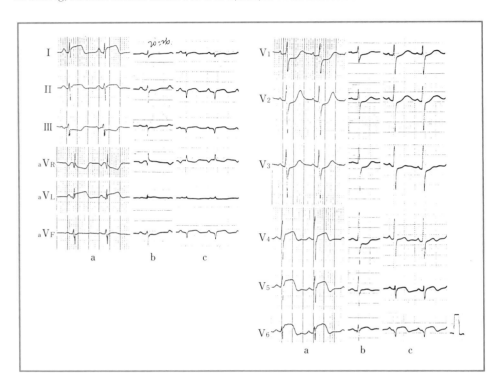

FIG. 436 Electrocardiograms. a: 54 days before death, at onset of infarct; b: 33 days before death, during chest pain; c: 30 days before death, after disappearance of chest pain.

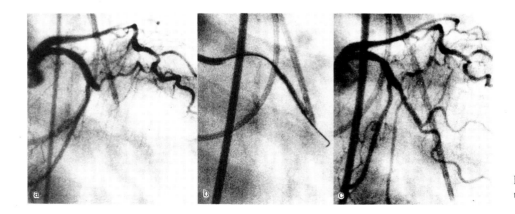

FIG. 437 PTCA. a: control; b: during dilation; c: after dilation.

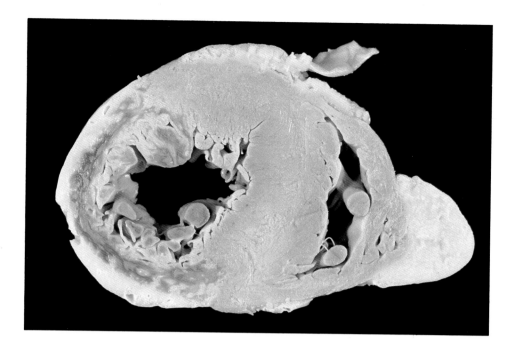

FIG. 438 Transverse section. Heart weight: 370 g. Translucent white fibrosis is present in the posterolateral wall of the left ventricle. Some reddish-brown areas of coagulation necrosis are also present.

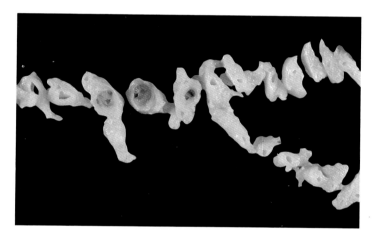

FIG. 439 Left coronary artery. Dilation of the stenotic region was achieved by dissociation of the intima, but thrombi are still present.

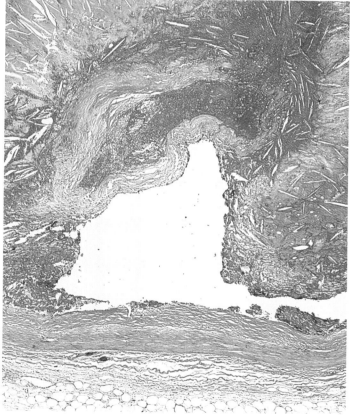

FIG. 440 Histologic findings in the left circumflex artery. A thrombus resulting from rupture of the atheroma and dilation of the lumen resulting from dissociation of the intima can be seen. (HE stain, × 43.)

CASE 31 PTCA (2)

The patient was a 64-year-old man who smoked 60 cigarettes a day. He was hypertensive but not diabetic. A thoracic aortic aneurysm was found 5 years before death. He was examined by a local physician because of hoarseness 6 months before death, and enlargement of the thoracic aortic aneurysm was noted. Four months before death, he was admitted. An anterior septal wall infarction occurred on the sixth day after admission. The serum CK was 581 IU/L. Left ventriculography and coronary angiography revealed 90% stenosis of segment 6 and segment 9 of the left anterior descending artery. PTCA was performed before surgery for the thoracic aortic aneurysm 85 days before death. Stenosis in segment 6 of the left anterior descending artery was improved to 43%. Bypass grafting was performed for the thoracic aortic aneurysm 58 days before death. Pneumonia occurred as a complication postoperatively and the patient died.

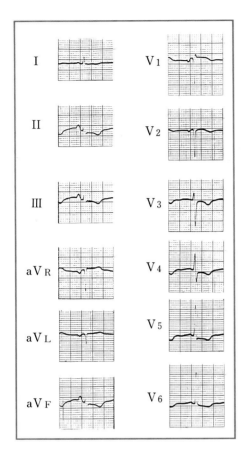

FIG. 441 Electrocardiograms at rest.

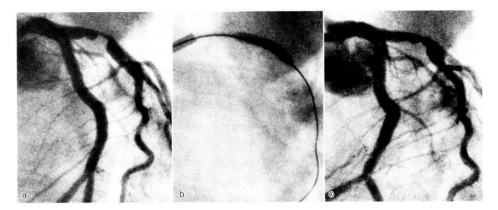

FIG. 442 PTCA. a: control; b: during dilation; c: after dilation.

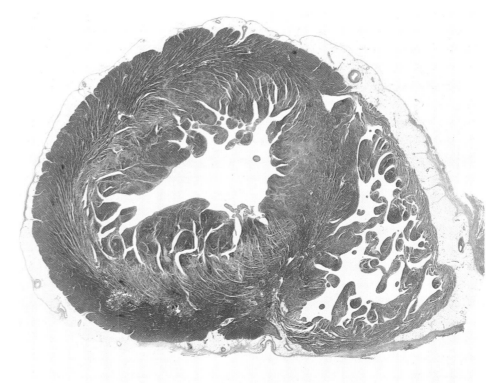

FIG. 443 Histologic transverse section. Small areas of fibrosis are evident in the anterior portion of the interventricular septum and anterior wall of the left ventricle. (Masson trichrome stain.)

11. Coronary Artery Bypass Grafting

Coronary artery bypass grafting (CABG) is a surgical technique designed to improve the blood supply to ischemic myocardium by bypassing stenotic or occluded regions of the coronary arteries. The objectives of CABG are (1) to improve angina pectoris, (2) to improve left ventricular function and motility, and (3) to prevent myocardial infarction.

Conventionally, CABG mainly required use of the great saphenous vein, but there is a recent trend toward increasing use of arterial grafts from the internal mammalian and gastroepiploic arteries to improve long-term patency.

Luminal stenosis associated with intimal hypertrophy of venous grafts used for CABG is of clinical pathologic importance. The prophylaxis of intimal thickening and stenosis are the most important factors affecting the long-term CABG performance. Table 12 summarizes the time course of histopathologic changes in venous grafts compiled from autopsy cases.

Although little intimal hypertrophy is seen in cases 1 year or more postoperatively, after 3 years or longer, atherosclerosis may gradually progress, leading to intimal stenosis. Therefore, changes in venous grafts apparently occur by the same mechanism as atherosclerosis of the arterial system.

Table 12. Time course of histopathologic findings in great saphenous vein grafts

Period until death	Main findings	
	Intima	**Media and adventitia**
Intraoperatively, postoperatively, or at least 1 day postoperatively	Small numbers of erythrocytes and leukocytes, small amounts of fibrin deposition	None
1 week postoperatively	Increase in fibrin	Mild edema of media
1 month postoperatively	Increases in smooth muscle cells and collagen	Necrosis of media
6 months postoperatively	Incorporation of fibrin in the intima Appearance of foam cells → intimal hypertrophy	Fibrosis of both media and adventitia
1 year postoperatively	Fibrous intimal hyperplasia	Fibrosis
>1 year postoperatively	Intimal hypertrophy stops or atherosclerosis appears after 3 years	

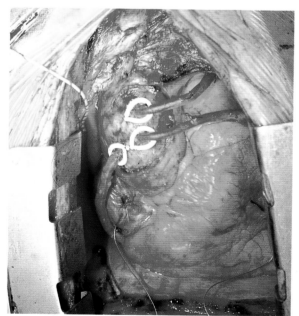 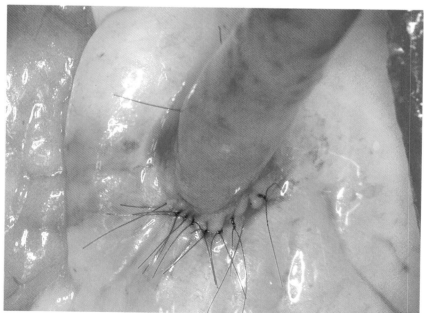

FIG. 454 Photographs at operation of coronary artery bypass grafting using the great saphenous vein. The left figure shows the central anastomosis between the origin of the aorta and the great saphenous vein graft. The right figure shows the peripheral anastomosis between the great saphenous vein and the coronary arteries.

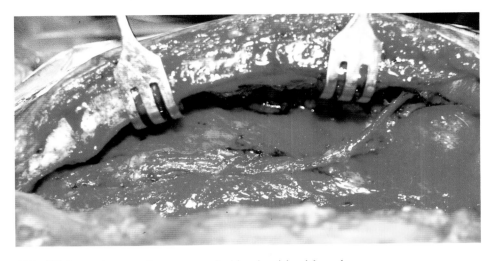

FIG. 455 Internal mammalian artery graft ablated and freed from the thoracic wall.

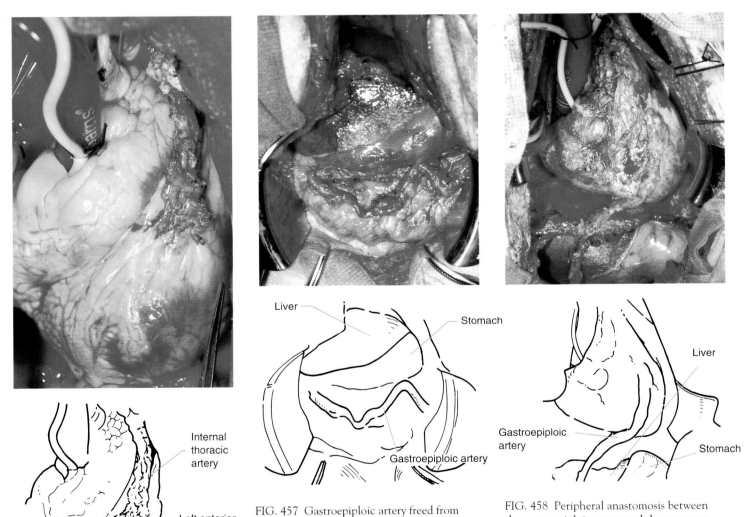

FIG. 456 Peripheral anastomosis of the internal thoracic artery and the left anterior descending artery.

FIG. 457 Gastroepiploic artery freed from the stomach.

FIG. 458 Peripheral anastomosis between the gastroepiploic artery and the coronary artery.

Case 33 Coronary Artery Bypass Grafting (1)

The patient was a 55-year-old woman who was hypertensive and diabetic. Angina pectoris on effort began about 5 years before death, and she was admitted 4 years 9 months before death for detailed investigation. Left ventriculography and coronary angiography revealed 75% stenosis of segment 6, 90% stenosis of segment 7, and 75% stenosis of segment 8 of the left anterior descending artery, 75% stenosis of segment 11 of the left circumflex artery, and 99% stenosis of segment 2 and 75% stenosis of segment 4 of the right coronary artery. Slightly weakened contraction was noted in the anterior basal and anterolateral walls, apex, diaphragm surface, and posterior basal and posterior walls, and the ejection fraction was 53%. Coronary artery bypass grafting (venous graft to the first diagonal branch, seg-

ment 8 of the left anterior descending artery, and the posterolateral branch) was performed 4 years 7 months before death. An inferoposterior wall transmural infarction occurred postoperatively. Postoperative angiography revealed complete occlusion of segment 7 of the left anterior descending artery, occlusion of the bypass to segment 8, and patency of the bypass to the first diagonal branch and posterolateral branch. The ejection fraction was 46%. Thereafter, angina pectoris developed. Exertional dyspnea began about 1 month before death. The patient was admitted because of heart failure 6 months before death, and acute occlusion of the superior mesenteric artery occurred 2 months before death. An inferior wall myocardial infarction developed on the same day, the patient's general condition deteriorated, and she died.

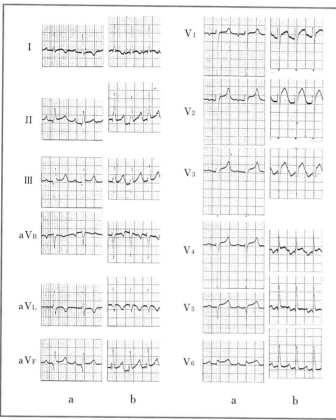

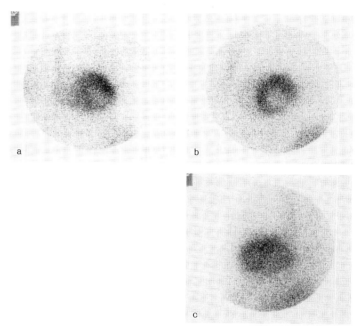

FIG. 460 Myocardial scintigrams. a: frontal surface; b: left anterior oblique 45° aspect; c: lateral surface. A defect image resulting from postoperative infarction can be seen in the inferoposterior wall after coronary artery bypass grafting.

FIG. 459 Electrocardiograms. a: day of death; b: 1 day before death.

FIG. 461 Left ventriculography. a: end-diastole; b: end-systole.

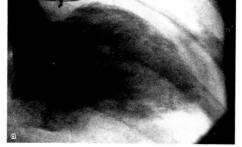

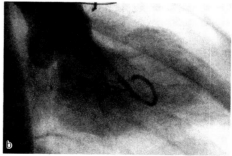

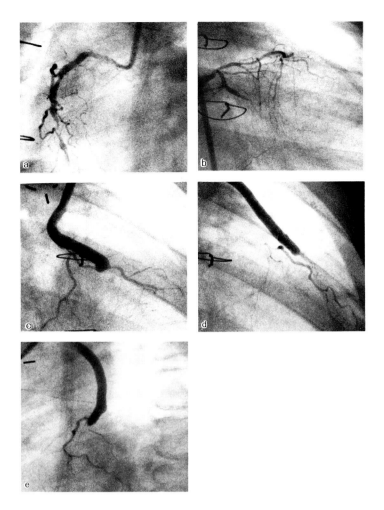

FIG. 462 Coronary angiography. Postoperative angiography, a: right coronary artery; b: left coronary artery; c: venous graft to the obtuse marginal branch; d: graft to the left anterior descending artery; e: graft to the diagonal branch.

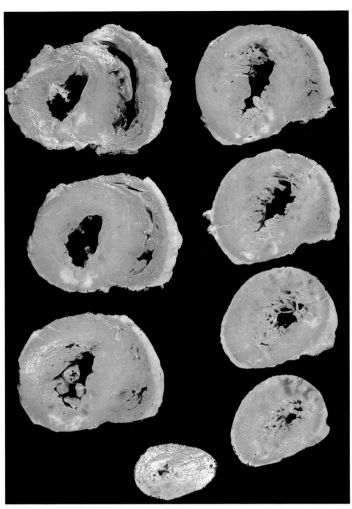

FIG. 464 Transverse sections. White fibrosis is seen in the posterior wall of the left ventricle. Discoloration is present in the anterior wall of the left ventricle near the apex.

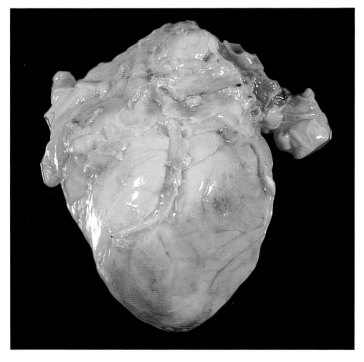

FIG. 463 Frontal surface of the heart. Heart weight: 550 g. The great saphenous vein graft to the left anterior descending artery is shown. The epicardium shows fibrous adhesion.

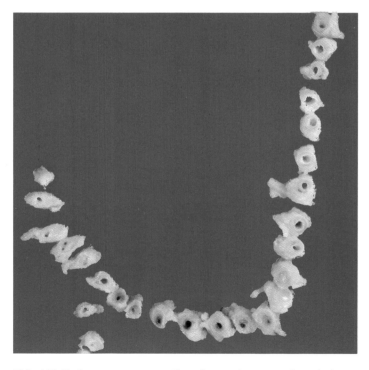

FIG. 465 Right coronary artery. Complete occlusion resulting from an atheroma is evident in the distal part.

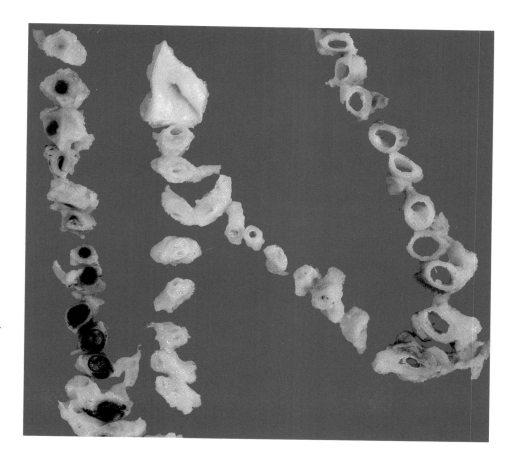

FIG. 466 Right coronary artery and bypass. The left anterior descending artery shows severe stenosis of more than 90% in the proximal part, and the bypass to the left anterior descending artery is occluded by a thrombus. The left circumflex artery is almost completely occluded in the proximal part. The bypass to the posterolateral branch is open, but fibrous hypertrophy can be noted in the intima.

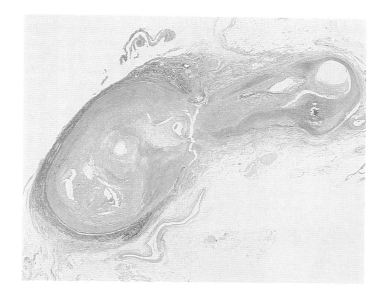

FIG. 467 Histologic findings in the peripheral anastomosis of the bypass of the left anterior descending artery. The bypass shows intimal thickening associated with an atheroma and is almost completely occluded. (Elastica van Gieson stain, × 12.5.)

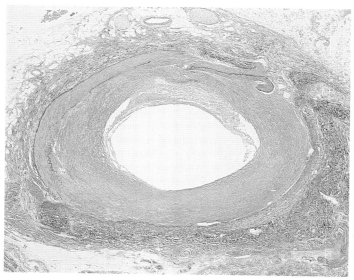

FIG. 468 Histologic findings in the peripheral anastomosis of the bypass to the posterolateral branch of the left coronary artery. Fibrous intimal thickening is evident in the coronary artery and the bypass. (Elastica van Gieson stain, × 21.)

CASE 34 CORONARY ARTERY BYPASS GRAFTING (2)

The patient was a 64-year-old man who smoked 40 cigarettes a day. He was hypertensive but not diabetic. Angina pectoris on effort appeared 5 years 1 month before death. He was admitted to a local hospital because of a myocardial infarction 4 years 4 months before death. Chest pain persisted thereafter, and 3 years 10 months before death the patient was hospitalized for a detailed examination. Left ventriculography and coronary angiography revealed 90% stenosis of segment 4 of the right coronary artery, 75% stenosis of segment 5 of the left coronary artery, 90% stenosis of segment 6 of the left anterior descending artery, and 75% stenosis of segment 11 and 90% stenosis of segment 12 of the left circumflex artery. No contraction was seen in the apex and diaphragmatic surface. The cardiac index was 3.0 L/min/m². Coronary artery bypass grafting (segment 8 of the left anterior descending artery and the posterolateral branch of the right coronary artery) was performed. Angina pectoris resolved, but recurred 9 months before death. He was admitted to the coronary care unit (CCU) 45 days before death as a result of persistence of severe angina pectoris. Coronary angiography revealed complete occlusion of segment 1 of the right coronary artery, 75% stenosis of segment 5 of the left coronary artery, complete occlusion of segments 6 and 8 and 99% stenosis of segment 9 of the left anterior descending artery, 90% stenosis of segment 11, and complete occlusion of segment 12 of the left circumflex artery. The bypass to the left anterior descending artery showed 50% stenosis at the anastomosis. The bypass to the posterolateral branch of the right coronary artery was occluded at the origin. A Killip I infarction occurred in the posterolateral wall 35 days before death. The maximum serum CK was 1,782 IU/L and maximum SGOT 344 IU/L. Thereafter, anginal attacks continued. A Killip II and Forrester III lateral wall infarction occurred 8 days before death. The maximum CK activity was 613 IU/L. The patient's general condition deteriorated, leading to death.

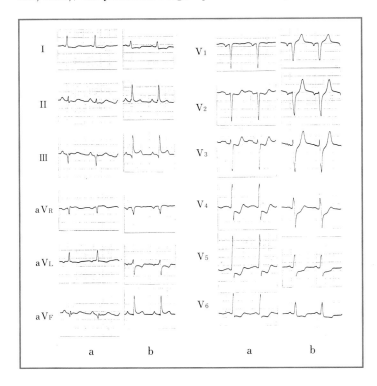

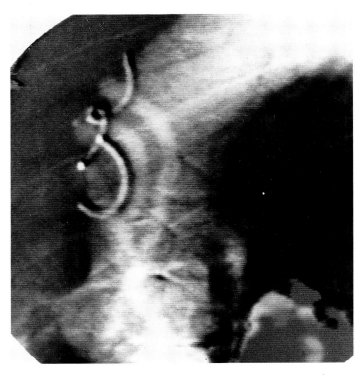

FIG. 469 Electrocardiograms. a: 45 days before death, during chest pain; b: 1 day before death, during onset of infarction.

FIG. 470 Digital subtraction angiography. Patency of the bypass graft was confirmed after coronary artery bypass surgery.

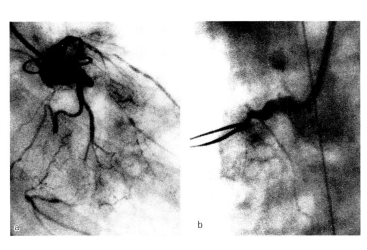

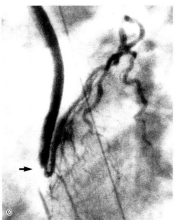

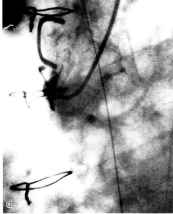

FIG. 471 Coronary angiography. a: left coronary artery; b: right coronary artery; c: venous graft to the left anterior descending artery; d: orifice of right coronary artery bypass graft.

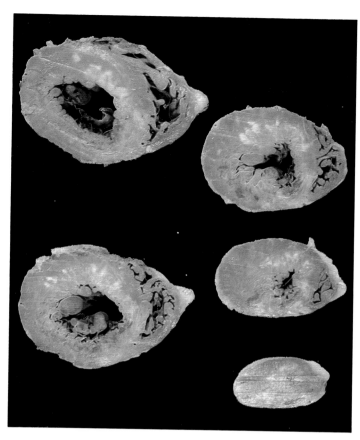

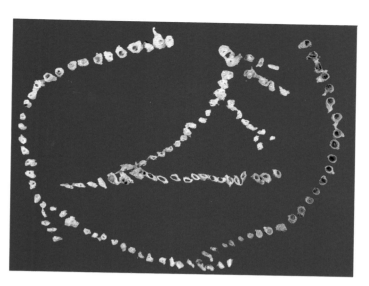

FIG. 473 Coronary arteries. Severe atheromatous stenosis of more than 90% was noted in the proximal parts of the right coronary artery and left anterior descending artery. The left circumflex artery shows hypoplasia. The graft to the left anterior descending artery is patent, but the bypass to the posterolateral branch of the right coronary artery shows atherosclerotic and thrombotic occlusion.

FIG. 472 Transverse sections. Heart weight: 440 g. White fibrosis is evident subendocardially in the anterior wall of the left ventricle and anterior portion of the interventricular septum. Translucent discoloration is observed subendocardially in the posterior wall.

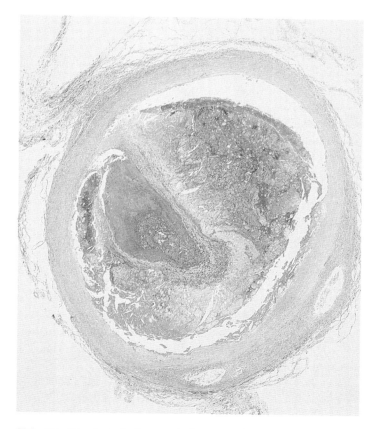

FIG. 474 Histologic findings in the bypass to the posterolateral branch of the right coronary artery. Rupture of the atheroma and thrombus are seen. (Masson trichrome stain, × 21.)

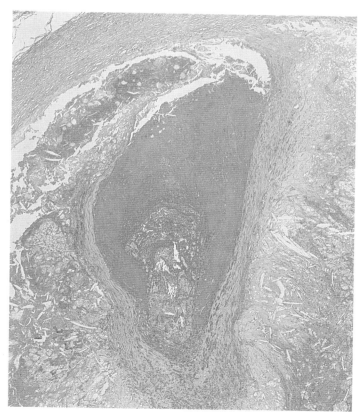

FIG. 475 Histologic findings in the bypass to the posterolateral branch of the right coronary artery. A marked atheroma is seen and the lumen is occluded by a thrombus. (HE stain, × 43.)

Suggested Readings

Internal Medicine

1. Killip T, Kimball JT: Treatment of myocardial infarction in a coronary care unit. Am J Cardiol 20:457, 1967

2. AHA Committee Report: A reporting system on patients evaluated for coronary artery disease. Circulation 51:5, 1975

3. Forrester JS, Diamond GA, Swan HJC: Correlative classification of clinical and hemodynamic function after acute myocardial infarction. J Cardiol 39:137, 1977

4. Gruentzig AR, Stenning A, Wiegenthaler WE: Non-operative dilatation of coronary artery stenosis. N Engl J Med 301:61, 1979

5. Rentrop P, Blanke H, Koestering K, Karsch KR: Acute myocardial infarction: intracoronary application of nitroglycerin and streptokinase in combination with transluminal recanalization. Clin Cardiol 5:354, 1979

6. Grossman W: Cardiac Catheterization and Angiography. 2nd Ed. Lea & Febiger, Philadelphia, 1980

7. Kimata S, Momma K, Inoue Y: Shinzo Dai Kekkan Zoei [Cardiac-macrovascular Angiography]. Igaku–shoin, Tokyo, 1981

8. Haze K, Hiramori K: Ushitsu Kosoku: Sono Byotai, Shindan, Chiryo [Right ventricular infarction: its pathology, diagnosis, and treatment]. Respir Circ 31:829, 1983

9. Haze K, Sumiyoshi T, Fukami K et al: Clinical characteristics of coronary artery spasm: electrocardiographic, hemodynamic and arteriographic assessment. Jpn Circ J 49:82, 1985

10. National Cardiovascular Center: Junkanki Shikkan No Chiryo Shishin [Treatment Strategies of Cardiovascular Diseases]. Maruzen, Tokyo, 1987

11. Braunwald W: Heart Disease. 3rd Ed. WB Saunders, Philadelphia, 1988

12. Haze K: p. 719. In Kameyama M et al (eds): Shinkinkosokusho, Kon–Getsu No Shindan Shishin [Myocardial Infarction, Diagnosis Strategies]. Igaku–shoin, Tokyo, 1988

13. Nobuyoshi M: [PTCA.] Igaku–shoin, Tokyo, 1988

14. Hiramori K, Saito M, Haze K (eds): Kan Domyaku Shikkan No Shuchu Chiryo [Intensive Care of Coronary Disease]. 3rd Ed. Nanko–do, Tokyo, 1989

Radiology

15. Strauss HW, Pitt B (eds): Cardiovascular Nuclear Medicine. 2nd Ed. CV Mosby, St Louis, 1979

16. Higgins CB: CT of the Heart and the Great Vessel. Futura Publishing, New York, 1983

17. Berman PS, Mason DT (eds): Clinical Nuclear Cardiology. Grune & Stratton, Orlando, FL, 1981

18. Inagaki Y, Masuda Y: Shin Dai Kekkan No CT Shindan [CT Diagnosis of Cardiac and Macrovascular Systems]. Igaku–shoin, Tokyo, 1984

19. Kaku Jiki Kyomei Igaku Kenkyu Kai [Medical NMR Association] (ed): NMR Igaku: Kiso To Rinsho [Medical NMR: Basic and Clinical Studies]. Maruzen, Tokyo, 1984

20. Nishimura T: Shinzo Kaku Igaku No Rinsho [Clinical Cardiac Nuclear Medicine]. Nagai–shoten, Osaka, 1984

21. Hoshasen Igaku Taikei Tokubekkan 2 [Medical Radiology Suppl 2]: Kaku Jiki Kyomei Gazo Shindan [Diagnosis of NMR Imaging]. Nakayama–shoten, Tokyo, 1987

22. Kozuka T, Hiramatu K (eds): DSA [Digital Subtraction Angiography]. Igaku–shoin, Tokyo, 1987

23. Nishimura T, Yonekura Y (eds): Atarashii Shinzo Kaku Igaku [Modern Cardiac Nuclear Medicine]. Kanehara, Tokyo, 1988

24. Stark DD, Bradley WG (eds): Magnetic Resonance Imaging. CV Mosby, St Louis, 1988

25. Nagai T (ed): MRI Shindan Gaku: Kiso To Rinsho [MRI Diagnosis: Basic and Clinical Studies]. Asakura, Tokyo, 1989

26. Nishimura T (ed): Shinkin SPECT Zufu [Myocardial SPECT Imaging]. Nagai–shoten, Osaka, 1989

Ultrasound

27. Machii K (ed): Danso Shin Echo Zu [Cardiac Echo Tomography]. Chugai Igaku, Tokyo, 1981

28. Nimura Y, Machii K, Kato H (eds): Rinsho Danso Shin Echo Zu Handoku Koza [Seminar for the Clinical Diagnosis of Cardiac Echo Tomography]. Kanehara, Tokyo, 1982

29. Omoto R (ed): Real Time Doppler Danso Shin Echo Zu Ho [Real-time Doppler Cardiac Echo Tomography]. Shindan To Chiryo, Tokyo, 1983

30. Nanda NC: Doppler Echocardiography. Igaku-shoin, New York, 1985

31. Chikai T, Matsuo H (eds): Cho Onpa Igaku [Medical Ultrasound]. Nagai–shoten, Osaka, 1985

32. Feigenbaum H: Echocardiography. 4th Ed. Lea & Febiger, Philadelphia, 1986

33. Kitabatake A, Inoue M (eds): Cho Onpa Shinzo Doppler Ho [Cardiac Doppler Ultrasound]. Maruzen, Tokyo, 1986

34. Yoshikawa J (ed): Cho Onpa Doppler Ho No Rinsho [Doppler Ultrasound in Practice]. Medical Core, 1986

35. Hoshasen Igaku Taikei [Clinical Radiology]: Cho Onpa Shindan (I) [Ultrasound Diagnosis (I)]. Nakayama–shoten, Tokyo, 1988

36. Kozuka T (ed): Shinzo No Gazo Shindan [Diagnosis of Cardiac Imaging]. Maruzen, Tokyo, 1988

Pathology

37. Gould SE: Pathology of the Heart and Blood Vessels. 3rd Ed. Charles C Thomas, Springfield, 1968

38. Pomerance A, Davies MJ: The Pathology of the Heart. Blackwell Scientific Publications, Oxford, England, 1975

39. Crawford T: Pathology of Ischemic Heart Disease. Butterworths, London, 1977

40. Netter FH: Heart: The Ciba Collection of Medical Illustrations. Vol. V. CIBA, New York, 1978

41. Rossi L: Histopathology of Cardiac Arrhythmias. Casa Editrica Ambrosiano, Milano, Italy, 1978

42. Olsen EGJ: The Pathology of the Heart. 2nd Ed. Macmillan Press, London, 1980

43. Horie T: Shikin Kosoku [Myocardial Infarction]. Igaku-shoin, Tokyo, 1981

44. Becker AE, Anderson RH: Cardiac Pathology. Gower Medical Publishing, New York, 1982

45. Sugiura M, Okawa S: Ronenki Shinzobyo No Rinsho To Byori [Clinical Pathology of Heart Disease in Geriatric Patients]. Nanko–do, Tokyo, 1982

46. Silver MD: Cardiovascular Pathology. Churchill Livingstone, New York, 1983

47. Davies MJ: Cardiovascular Pathology. Harvey Miller, Oxford University Press, London, 1986

48. Olsen EGJ: Cardiovascular Pathology. MTP Press, Lancaster, England, 1987

49. Yutani C, Ishibashi-Ueda H, Konishi M et al: Histopathological study of acute myocardial infarction and pathoetiology of coronary thrombosis: a comparative study in districts in Japan. Jpn Circ J 51:352, 1987

50. Hurst JW, Anderson RH, Becker AE, Wilcox BR: Atlas of the Heart. Gower Medical Publishing, New York, 1988

51. Kawasaki T, Shigemitu I, Hamashima Y et al: Kawasaki Byo [Kawasaki Disease]. Nanko–do, Tokyo, 1988

52. Nobuyoshi M: Rinsho Shinzo Catheter Ho [Clinical Cardiac Catheter Report]. Igaku-shoin, Tokyo, 1988

53. Waller BF (ed): Contemporary Issues in Cardiovascular Pathology. FA Davis, Philadelphia, 1988

54. Waller BF (ed): Pathology of the Heart and Great Vessels. Churchill Livingstone, New York, 1988

55. Okada R, Kawai Y: Color Atlas Shinkin Kosoku [Color Atlas of Myocardial Infarction]. Boehringer-Ingerheim Japan, Hyogo, 1989

56. Hashimoto M, Ohtsu M, Iijima S: Color Atlas Shin Shikkan 100 Rei [Color Atlas of 100 Cases of Heart Disease]. Dainippon Seiyaku, Osaka, 1989

57. Schoen FJ: Interventional and Surgical Cardiovascular Pathology. WB Saunders, Philadelphia, 1989

58. Yutani C, Imakita M, Ishibashi-Ueda H: Histopathological study of aorto-coronary bypass grafts with special reference to fibrin deposits on grafted saphenous veins. Acta Pathol Jpn 39:425, 1989

Surgery

59. Kalsner S: The Coronary Artery. Croom Helm, London, 1982

60. Mason D, Collins JJ: Myocardial Revascularisation. York Medical Books, USA, 1982

61. Wheatley DJ: Surgery of Coronary Artery Disease. CV Mosby, St Louis, 1986